Take Care of Your Hair or You Might Lose It Like me!

DISCLAIMER

This e-book has been written for information purposes only. Every effort has been taken towards making this e-book as true, complete and accurate as possible. However, there may be mistakes in typography or content. Also, this e-book provides information relevant to taken care of the hair only up to the publishing date. Therefore, this e-book should be used as a guide – knowing that new information are constantly coming up.

The purpose of this e-book is to educate. The author and the publisher do not warrant that the information contained in this e-book is fully complete and shall not be responsible for any errors or omissions. The author and publisher shall have neither liability nor responsibility to any person or entity with respect to any loss or damage caused or alleged to be caused directly or indirectly by this e-book.

COPYRIGHT

Take Care of Your Hair or You Might Lose It Like me!

Copyright © 2015

DEDICATION

This book is dedicated to our beloved readers whose quests for knowledge knows no bound

They have inspired me to create this e-book to be a helpful tool for them and the millions out there.

Happy reading.

FOREWORD

It is indeed with a great sense of pleasure and privilege that I give this foreword to the book *Take Care of Your Hair or You Might Lose It Like me!* written by Sabat Beatto and a team of experts who specializes in hair care and general body wellness.

Several readily understandable sections with *abstract* and *Keywords* have been included to make the subject comprehension and revision easy and fun. The approach utilized in dealing with the subject of hair care in this book will not only be enjoyed by readers alone but by other gurus in this field as well. I have no doubt that this will be a valuable addition to the life of any reader and will further strengthen the foundation of body care in particular and fashion in general.

Signature

Sabat Beatto

ACKNOWLEDGEMENTS

A special thanks to my dedicated members of staff for creating the title. Also acknowledged are other specialists in the department of body care.

I will not forget my many friends, clients, readers who provided the opportunity to write this amazing book.

Thank you, all, you are appreciated.

Sabat Beatto

CONTENTS

INTRODUCTION

A Family Affair for Hair

Out of the hundreds of procedures he performs each year, the last thing hair-transplant surgeon Dr. Robert Dorin expected to do was perform surgery on his father. Robert M. Dorin Sr. had been losing his hair for many years now, but few people knew how much it bothered him. Then, one day at a family function, the elder Dorin casually mentioned to his son that he was considering treatment.

"It surprised me because my father knew what type of work I do and he never said anything," Dorin said.

Caught unawares, Dorin was nevertheless delighted that his father was taking matters into his own hands.

 "My father's hair loss finally reached a point where most of the hair in the frontal area had fallen out," he said.

So Dorin decided to come up with a surprise of his own.

"Given that it was a week before my dad's birthday, I figured it was a great opportunity to give him a gift that he would enjoy for the rest of his life," he said. "I scheduled a procedure for my father for the very next week."

On the day of the surgery, the two discussed the details of the procedure and what to expect.

"I could feel and see my dad's excitement grow as things took shape," Dorin said. "He realized just how much hair he had lost over the years and how much I would be able to put back in just one procedure."

The procedure required 1,571 hair-transplant grafts and took about 7 hours. Three weeks later, there were no telltale signs of the hair transplant. He should begin enjoying his new look in three to six months.

"Working on my dad was something extra special for me, it was an honor to be able to do something that would have a lasting, positive impact on his life. It is very similar to the way his actions and support have shaped my life." Dorin concluded.

Arresting the Age Old Problem of Hair Loss

Men aren't the only ones looking for a cure for hair loss. Some women are also affected. One solution is delving into the Internet for answers. Cyberspace will provide you with a number of solutions to this confidence-breaking problem. You can even sift through a variety of reviews posted by individuals who have tried specific products.

Depending on what you're willing to spend, there is surely a hair loss cure suitable to you. I recall when my older brother Christopher began losing his dew towards the end of high school. I felt awkward about this I must admit. Why do some guys start losing their hair at such a tender age? Much actually depends on genetics and stress. I'm guessing it was stress in this case since my mother's father has a full head of hair.

If you watch television, then you've most likely spotted a hair loss commercial or two. Those sometimes quirky, yet cheesy ads don't offer much solace when we start going bald up top or the forehead starts to expand. Luckily there are quality solutions at hand. The first step you should take concerning a cure for hair loss is consulting a family doctor or possibly a trichologist. He or she will be able to present you with some decent options.

The good news is many of these products are effective, and not so expensive these days. You can get your hair back. You just need to exhaust your resources in order to pinpoint that perfect cure for hair loss.

This certainly is the simplest choice, but it doesn't have to be your only option. You can find an effective cure for hair loss if you do your homework. In the cosmetically advanced world we currently reside in, there's no reason why you have to take your hair loss like a man.

Are you in desperate search of a cure for hair loss? Many men across the world are going through a daily struggle with hair loss. The inevitable affliction sadly becomes a reality for many of us. Although most men do not prefer a bald scalp, some are taking this route and avoiding the struggle altogether.

This can be helpful in your search for the right and ideal cure for hair loss. You've simply got to love the Internet. If you discover an over-the-counter cure for hair loss, you can likely pick it up at any corner drug store.

CHAPTER ONE

HAIR BASICS

Cycle of Hair Growth and Information on Follicles

Keywords: Hair cycle, hair growth, hair follicles, anagen, catagen, tologen, medical.

Abstract: Hair Grows At a rate of 1cm. per month and grow in a cycle consisting of 3 steps. The Follicles produce the hair and are replenished throughout the life of the human being. The time of phases of growth of the hair is determined genetically.

Hair Growth Rate and Cycle

At any Stage of our life, only 10% of hair is in resting phase. They Fall off in 2-3 months and the new hair grows in a total time of 2-6 years. About 90% of the hair grows on our scalp at a time and they grow at a rate of 1 cm. per month.

Normally hair lasts for two to four years in men and four to six years in Women.

How Hair Grows

Deep inside the hair follicle, the hair forms inside a hair bulb, protrude and grow outside.

Any Method of hair improvements like shampooing, conditioning, cutting, sun exposure does not affect the rate of growth of the hair.

There are 3 phases of hair growth:

- *Anagen* which takes a time of about 1000 days or 3 years.
- *Catagen* lasting for 10 days.
- *Tologen* for nearly 3 months.

Anagen includes the start of growth of hair and *Tologen* is the end i.e. the shedding phase of hair. The Hair bulb keeps on coming outside from the start to the shedding phase. Hair growth is effected by the seasonal changes, i.e. hair grows quicker in winter than in summer as a result of the seasonal change. In the *Catagen* phase, hair growth is stopped for a small time and no pigment is produced at this time.

The time of *Anagen* Phase is usually fixed and is determined genetically and is also responsible for the length of the hair. The no. of hair follicles in a human head counts approximately 100,000. Each Follicle produces hair for about 20 times in the lifetime. In a new born baby, the hair follicles grow hair in Unison, i.e. all at a same time but as time passes, the follicles produce hairs at different times.

If a hair is plucked from the head, the follicle is not ruptured but it starts to produce a new hair. As age increases, the shedding of follicles is evidently seen in most of the people in the top of the head and also in the forehead. The Hair does not grow in a definite straight manner but makes the follicle to stand in some constant angle. Depending on this angle, the hairs are always set to lie. The stream is usually in a twisted manner but it is then influenced by the way of combing of hair by people.

Finally, Hair grows at a slow rate, so utmost care is needed to prevent them from shedding.

Daily Hair Care

Your hair makes you look gorgeous, bold and beautiful. It is because of your hair that you attract the attention of other people. So it is natural that you will always expect that your hair will look good and in a way that people will like them. But certainly your hair didn't fulfill your expectations on every other day. Even though some time you feel disappointed because of your hair. The reason is simple; you are unable to keep them as you want and as others like them. In such a situation definitely, you would like to spend some time with your hair. It is obvious that you need to know about Hair Care.

But before jumping into those hair care tips it is equally important to know the factors which affects your hair and hairstyle?

Factors Affecting Hair and Hairstyle

The biologists argue that the characteristics of the hair of a person depend on several factors some of which are inherited. Some factors are genetic, meaning that DNA programming is responsible for your hairs; the way they look. The secretion level of hormones also contributes to hair looks. And after all, the entire environment especially the air and water greatly affects your hairstyle. That's why, every person some time experience the bad hair day. But if you are willing to take a little care, you can say goodbye to bad hair day, which might not be permanent and need your attention time to time.

Tips on Hair Care

Here are few tips that will help you to either not see a bad hair day or to come out if you are experiencing it at present:

- Stick to a healthy life style. Give up your smoking habits, do exercise regularly, eat balanced diet and use relaxation techniques when stressed.
- Get a deep sleep at night, do not sleep with burdens otherwise you will have a disturbed sleep enough to trap into a bad hair day.
- If you are using hair styling products and cosmetics, try to avoid using products containing alcohol particularly in high concentration.
- Do not put hair styling products on your scalps, this will block the pores on your head and may harm your head and hair both.

- Swimming is a good exercise, do it. But before jumping into a swimming pool wet your hair enough with plain water. Pool water contains chlorine, which is not good for your hair.
- Set your hair dryer on cool settings, hot is not good for your hair.
- Keep hair dryer moving, do not stick it to one place for long.
- Before using hair dryer, use a good quality towel to dry hair and then use hair dryer to get the rid of wetness.
- Use a comb that bristles are made of animal hairs, it would be soft on your hairs.
- Always use clean comb / brushes. Clean your comb / brushes with soap or shampoo on a regular basis.
- Always comb / brush your hair downwards.
- Shampooing your hair is important. Always use good quality products.
- Use trial and error method to select a shampoo for you and choose the one that is best suitable.

Hair Coloring

Keywords: Coloring hair, Hair coloring ideas, natural hair coloring, hair coloring ideas

Abstract: Coloring hair is very fashionable these days. You can easily see people of all age groups going for hair coloring. Hair coloring has been in use since the ancient times. Now-a-days, coloring hair is very much popular throughout the world.

History of Hair Coloring

Coloring hair is very fashionable these days. You can easily see people of all age groups going for hair coloring. People are experimenting with all kinds of colors to look fashionable. It is no longer just natural black or golden that people are going for, but they are experimenting with even red, green and blue and coming up with new hair coloring ideas.

Hair coloring has been in use since the ancient times. Ancient Greeks used to color or lighten their hair, which identified with honor and courage. They used harsh soaps to lighten or color their hair. There is evidence that ancient Romans also used to color or lighten their hair.

Now-a-days, coloring hair is very much popular throughout the world. According to some reports around 75% of women in the U.S. color their hair. Now people do not go for hair coloring just to hide their grey hair but to make a fashion statement as well. Young people are equally experimenting with many hair coloring ideas. The market for hair colors is huge and spreading all over the world.

Hair Coloring Products; how they work

There are many products for coloring hair available in the market. There are permanent as well as temporary colors. A patch test should be conducted before using any coloring product to see if the person is allergic to the color or not. In the case that the person is found allergic to chemicals used in hair colors, the use of the same should be stopped immediately.

Some people lighten their hair, which is also known as bleaching or decoloring. This process involves the diffusion of the natural color pigment or artificial coloring of the hair.

Permanent hair coloring products contain **oxidising agent** and an **alkalizing ingredient**. These chemicals raise the cuticle of the hair fibre so the color can penetrate in the hair fiber. They also facilitate the formation of tints within the hair fibre and bring about the lightening action of peroxide.

In the case of **temporary colors,** the pigment molecules are large so they do not penetrate the cuticle layer. It allows only a coating action that may be removed by shampooing. Temporary hair coloring products come in various forms like shampoos and gels.

Normally, temporary colors are used to give brighter colors to the hair. It is because temporary hair colorants do not penetrate the hair shaft itself. Instead, these dyes remain adsorbed to the follicle and can be easily removed with a single shampooing.

Hair Coloring can be damaging

The use of color can cause damage to hair in some cases. It is always better to visit an expert when you intend to undergo hair coloring to avoid any kind of harm done to the hair. Coloring hair in some cases can cause breakage of hair strands, hair fall and dry scalp.

CHAPTER TWO

CAUSES OF HAIR LOSS

Can Too Little Protein Cause Hair Loss?

Keywords: hair thinning, hair loss, hair, hair growth, fast hair growth, bald, balding, female hair loss, menopause.

Abstract: Hair usually grows about half an inch per month, although this slows as you age. Each hair remains on your head for two to six years, and during most of this time is continually growing. But many factors can disrupt this cycle. The result can be that your hair falls out early or isn't replaced.

Protein and Hair Loss

A new discovery has been made in finding out what actually causes hair loss, namely: the hardening of collagen. Persons who do not suffer from hair loss have supple collagen.

Hair usually grows about half an inch per month, although this slows as you age. Each hair remains on your head for two to six years, and during most of this time is continually growing. But many factors can disrupt this cycle. The result can be that your hair falls out early or isn't replaced.

A new discovery has been made in finding out what actually causes hair loss, namely: the hardening of collagen. Persons who do not suffer from hair loss have **supple collagen** and persons who begin showing signs of hair loss have **hardened collagen**. Collagen hardening interferes with the healthy functioning of the hair roots. The vital exchange process of the hair follicle cycle is disrupted and the hair becomes suffocated.

But What Causes Hair Loss?

Diet: Too little protein in your diet can lead to hair shedding, so can too little iron. Bottom line: Too strenuous dieting can result in hair loss! If you want to lose weight, do it the sensible way, especially if you have a hair thinning/loss problem to begin with.

Childbirth: Some women lose large amounts of hair within two to three months after delivery.

Hot Tips!

One great tip is after washing your hair, dry it in whatever manner you normally do. Then turn your head upside down, give your head a vigorous shake, and once back in a standing position, either "place" your hair using your fingers, rather than a brush or comb. You can also use a hair pick to style your hair. The upside down, shaking, also gives a great deal of fullness to otherwise flat looking thin hair. You'd be amazed at how creative you can be with your fingers without pulling at the root of the hair!

To protect your hair, the best practice is to shampoo only when hair is dirty. Because fine hair gets dirty faster, people with fine-textured hair need to shampoo more frequently -- even though fine hair breaks more easily. For that reason, fine-textured hair benefits from a good shampoo and volume-building conditioner

Biotin and Hair Loss

Keywords: Biotin, suffering hair problems, biotin deficiency, Biotin enriched shampoo, maintaining level of biotin, Sources of Biotin, Symptoms of Biotin Deficiency

Abstract: The e-book 'Biotin and Hair Loss' emphasizes on root cause of hair problems i.e. Biotin deficiency in the body. After reading this e-book you will be aware of hair problems and will be able to solve them with the help of experts. You will also become aware about properties of Biotin; a vitamin of B complex group sometime also known as vitamin H or vitamin B7.

The Importance of Biotin

Falling hair is normal, when you take your bath, roll on the bed, do combing and other such activities, you lose some of your hairs. It is very natural. But if your hair falls and that too in such a quantity that makes your head poor haired then it is a deficiency, which may ultimately lead to baldness. If this is the case, then you are suffering hair problems. The causes may be many and you need to identify them, but ultimately your body is deficient of Biotin. Yes, Biotin, is the vitamin, which makes your hair healthy, strong and good looking. It is clinically proven, so maintaining a good level of Biotin in your body system is as essential as maintaining other vitamins and minerals. Biotin is necessary for your hairs health and overall wellbeing. Medical specialists advise that the persons suffering with Hair Problems must take Biotin in addition to other medications.

So, if you are suffering hair problems, you must go for medications with Biotin substitutes. Foods like egg yolk and liver contains a lot of Biotin, you need to consume these foods in rich quantity to maintain your health and prevent hair loss.

Using a Biotin enriched shampoo may also help in improving your hair health.

Some more foods rich in Biotin are;

- Brewer's yeast,
- Green peas,
- Oats,
- Soybeans,
- Walnuts,
- Sunflower seeds,
- Bulgur and
- Brown rice, etc.

Eating these foods and other enriched food products will help your body in maintaining a good level of Biotin. A person who is a patient of heartburn, acid reflux or GERD absorbs less amount of Biotin, and hence may trap into hair problems. This is because; a person suffering with the above mentioned disease takes a lot of antacids.

So now, you will definitely agree with the fact that Biotin is a hair food, and important for good hair health.

What else does Biotin do for your body?

Biotin is a member of Vitamin B complex family also sometime known as Vitamin H or Vitamin B7. This is soluble in water, which means, if the body has a high level of Vitamin H at a certain day or time, it passes out through the urine. This vitamin is produced in the intestine with the help of the bacteria in the intestine. Biotin helps in the metabolism of carbohydrates, fats and proteins and helps in maintaining steady blood sugar. So, it is good for the persons suffering with Diabetes. Diabetes is a major disease across the globe and affects several men and women.

Biotin does the processing of glucose and we know glucose is one of the sources of energy for our body to perform work and maintain wear and tear of the body. Biotin also helps in the making of DNA, RNA and nucleic acids and production of fatty acids. Growth and replication of cells also depends on Biotin.

Thus on one hand Biotin helps in maintaining good hair health and on the other hand it is important for several bodily functions.

Sources of Biotin

The main sources of Biotin are; liver, kidneys, milk, cheese, butter and other dairy products, egg yolks, oysters, lobsters, poultry, cauliflower, avocados, bananas, strawberries, watermelon, grapefruits, raisins, mushrooms, green peas, blackcurrants, brewer's yeast, wheat germ, nuts, beans, lentils, oat bran, whole grains, oatmeal, peanut butter, molasses, and foods like salmon, tuna, mackerel, and herrings (foods rich in Omega – 3 fatty acids).

A healthy person and pregnant woman must take 300 grams of Biotin in daily diet. Breastfeeding mothers need about 350 micrograms of Biotin.

Symptoms of Biotin Deficiency

People affected with Biotin deficiency may show

- Dry or scaly scalp
- Loss of appetite
- Hair problems; closely associated with Biotin deficiency
- Nausea
- Depression
- Dermatitis
- Anorexia, and
- Anemia.

Andropause

Keywords: Andropause, male menopause, male menopause symptom, hair loss

Summary: Andropause and hair loss often go hand in hand. But there are plenty of things you can do to stop hair loss and promote healthy growth. Find out what you need to do now.

Andropause and Hair Loss

Andropause and hair loss often go hand in hand. Imagine clumps of hair falling off your head, or observing strands of once healthy hair collecting in the shower drain. Maybe you run your hand through your hair and feel it thinning. It can feel daunting and quite scary.

Typically, hair loss is a result of an imbalance of male testosterone hormone in the body. Instead of infusing the hair with healthy testosterone, enzymes break it down to a simpler form known as dihydrotestosterone.

An excess of this hormone has the effect of decreasing the size of hair follicles which eventually break down and make your hair fall off sporadically. The medical condition that is best associated with hair loss in Andropause sufferers is **hyperthyroidism**. Hyperthyroidism is a by-product of decreasing levels of Human Growth Hormone (HGH), which is responsible for regulating our aging process. Andropause sufferers' hormones have a profound effect on the rate and consistency of hair loss. Dihydrotestosterone (considered by medical circles as the strongest, most potent form of testosterone) is responsible for building and growing body hair in men (at normal levels - an excess causes hair degeneration.)

This includes body hair, pubic hair, head hair, armpit hair – any hair. DHT is directly produced in the skin, made to work by supporting enzymes that break it down for distribution throughout the body. DHT levels are present more in certain areas of the body than in others – explaining why we may have a full crop of hair on our heads and little bushes of hair on our chests and backs. Realize, women also have DHT in their bodies but produce less of it.

That explains why women don't have body hair. Case in point: an excess of DHT is prevalent in Andropause sufferers, explaining the reason for hair loss. The enzyme used to break down testosterone to dihydrotestosterone is ¨over activated¨ - working too hard and too fast.

This is the primary cause for this Andropausal condition. As mentioned above, dihydrotestosterone is present more in certain areas of the body than in others. For this reason, men's hair can fall into funny patterns. You know, the balding train station clerk you might have seen with more hair on his scalp than the top of his head. The shrinking of hair follicles as a result of the production of DHT is attributed to this.

How Hair Grows

How hair grows is a wondrous thing in itself that needs to be recognized. Typically, hair grows at a rate of a quarter inch every 2 weeks. Andropause sufferers have their ¨hair growth cycles¨ disrupted when there is erratic growth of some hair strands where ¨new¨ hair pushed ¨old¨ hair out. Because Andropause is a period of hormonal imbalance, a lack of hormonal stability and poor homeostasis (holistic balance) in the body pushes things out of whack.

If you want to maintain healthy strands of hair, one thing you can do is hit that stair climber machine fellas! Exercise reverses the aging process and may certainly reverse this symptom. There are also hair loss treatment products that can help you recapture your hair.

Secondary causes of hair loss in men suffering Andropause is **stress**. More specifically, stress raises the levels of cortisol and cortisone (known as stress hormones) in the body. Eating non-nutritional foods also speeds up hair loss.

Pretty much any activity that speeds up the aging process will speed up your hair loss.

Stay away from caffeinated drinks, fast foods, and cigarette smoking to keep running your hands through your thick mane longer. Participate in recreational activities to reduce stress and light up your life with a proper exercise regimen.

If you're suffering from this condition, don't let it affect you in the least bit! Andropause should not serve as a punishment – rather, a realization of a future for the better.

Common Causes of Hair Loss

Keywords: reasons for hair loss, hair loss reason, hair loss causes, causes of hair loss, hair loss types, hair loss.

Abstract: This e-book tells you about various reasons for hair loss. After reading this e-book you will be convinced that your problem is temporary and hence you would be able to find some of the best solution for your hair loss problems.

Hair Loss

It is very natural for a person to loss 50 to 100 hairs each day under the body's hair renewal process. But most of the people at least once in their lifetime suffer heavy hair loss. There may be various reasons behind this; like medication, chemotherapy, exposure to radiations and certain chemicals, nutritional and hormonal factors, thyroid disease, skin disease or stress, etc.

In most of the cases hair loss is temporary but in certain cases it may be permanent depending on the severity of disease. Some of the most common causes of hair loss are explained here:

Hormonal Causes

Hormones are stimulant to hair growth and causes hair loss problems. Hormones heavily affect our hair growth. These affect male as well as female hair health.

Hair thinning: This is one of the hormonal problems and affects both men and women. Hair thinning in male is specific and follows a pattern from the front through to the crown. Hair thinning in female does not follow any specific pattern.

Hair thinning is caused by androgen DHT or dihydrotesterone. Everyone has DHT but only some suffers with hair problem. You are wandering, why? This is dependent on the hair follicles, which have a greater number of androgen receptors for the DHT to attach with. Till date, the most effective treatment for the problems of hair thinning is; anti-androgens. Anti-androgens are preventive drugs that prevent the creation of DHT. In future we may get genes therapy for hair thinning problems.

Childbirth: Many of the females experience hair loss after labor. In such a situation many of the hair enters the telogen or resting phase. Some of the females experiences hair loss within two to three months after giving childbirth.

Hair problem due to pregnancy is temporary, and in many of the cases, eradicate within time, say 1 to 6 months. This occurs because of diverse hormonal changes that take place within the body during pregnancy.

Birth control pills: Females who are genetically programmed with androgenic alopecia encounters hair loss at a much younger age when they takes birth control pills. Androgenic alopecia is caused due to various hormonal changes.

The females who have a history of hair loss in their family must consult doctors before taking any birth control pills. This type of hair loss is temporary and may stop in 1 to 6 months. But in some of the cases, it has been noticed that a female cannot regrow some of her hair that was lost due to Androgenic alopecia.

Deficient Diet

A good balanced diet rich in varied variety of nutrients is equally important to your hair health. The person who eats less of proteins or has irregular eating habits is liable to suffers hair loss. Generally to save protein our body pushes growing hair into resting phase. If your hair can be pulled out by the root very easily, then this may be due to lack of a well-balanced diet. This condition can be prevailed by eating a diet rich in proteins and other necessary nutrients.

Low Serum Iron

If some persons either may not have access to iron rich food or his / her body may not absorb enough iron, then this may cause hair problems. Women during menstrual period are more prone to be iron deficient. Low iron in the body can be detected by laboratory test and can be corrected by taking a diet rich in iron and iron pills.

Disease or Illness

Hair loss due to some disease or illness is very common, but this type of hair loss is temporary and lost hair may grow again. Diseases like sever infection or flu and high fever, thyroid disease etc may lead to hair loss. Certain medications, cancer treatments, and chronic illnesses also cause hair loss. A person who receives surgery also faces hair loss problems.

However, hair loss problems of any sort are generally temporary and can be solved by taking good nutritious diet and seeking professional help.

Alopecia and other Hair Loss Causes

Keywords: Hair loss, baldness, alopecia

Abstract: This e-book challenges the perception that baldness cannot be treated, offering hope to many sufferers. It focuses on the importance of determining the true causes of hair loss and seeking professional advice before embarking on a suitable course of treatment.

The Danger of Self Diagnosis and Treatment

One of the most worrying aspects of hair loss treatment is the tendency of so many people to seek solutions without first determining what caused their hair loss in the first place.

At best, sufferers may waste money on inappropriate 'wonder cures' or even legitimate treatments that unfortunately are not suitable for their particular needs. At worst, some people may be risking their health by self-prescribing powerful pharmaceutical drugs. I don't have a problem with hair loss sufferers saving money by purchasing cheap generic drugs on the internet, but I feel strongly that they should at least seek confirmation from their physician about whether a given drug matches their individual needs.

Hair Growth Cycle

Before examining the most common causes of premature hair loss we need to understand that some shedding of hair is perfectly normal. Hairs grow from follicles that are tiny organs in the skin designed to grow a single hair that follows this repetitive cycle:

1. **Lengthy Growth Period** (Anagen Stage) - this phase usually lasts between two and seven years with an average growth rate of six inches (15cm) each year.
2. **Short Transition Period** (Catagen Stage) - this period of transition lasts for roughly two to four weeks. During this phase, the hair shaft becomes detached and moves upwards within the follicle.
3. **Resting period** (Telogen Stage) - this phase lasts about three months allowing the hair to detach itself prior to falling out.

At this point a new hair begins to grow thus repeating the normal cycle of hair growth. Unfortunately a number of factors can interfere with the natural hair growth process leading to forms of hair thinning or premature baldness.

Common Causes of Hair Loss

Androgenetic alopecia is the most common cause of hair loss, probably accounting for as much as 95% of pattern hair loss for both men and women. It is usually associated with aging and develops in predictable stages over varying periods of time. Each follicle follows a genetically programmed growth cycle with some follicles coded to remain active for a shorter time than others. This results in the development of the hereditary baldness patterns that are so familiar to us all.

For this type of baldness to occur, the following factors must be present:

- A genetic predisposition for hair loss to occur (as explained above).
- The presence of male hormones.
- Aging - in other words, enough time for the first two factors to exert an influence.

All men and women produce male hormones such as testosterone and DHT. These have a useful role to play in both sexes but obviously occur in widely differing concentrations. It is the higher levels of androgens found in males that explains why this form of hair loss affects men more than women.

In brief, these hormones affect the hair growth cycle as follows:

- High levels of the 5-alpha-reductase enzyme occur in some cells of the hair follicle and sebaceous glands.
- 5-alpha-reductase converts testosterone into DHT.
- DHT causes the terminal hairs to miniaturize.
- This leaves short, soft, fluffy vellus hairs that provide inadequate scalp coverage.
- The growth phases gradually become shorter until these hairs are lost for good.

Alopecia areata - is thought to be an immune system disorder that causes follicles to stop producing hairs in patches on the head. In severe cases it can advance to the stage where all hair on the head is lost (*Alopecia totalis*) or even a complete absence of body hair results (*Alopecia universalis*).

In most cases the hair will reappear on its own but until then, the condition can be very distressing to sufferers particularly as its cause can be difficult to determine. If you feel you may be suffering from this form of hair loss, seek the advice of your physician who will carry out a physical examination and conduct blood tests to help determine the cause.

Telogen effluvium - is characterized by a general thinning or shedding of hair over a period of months and is most commonly found in people who have recently experienced trauma. Common causes include childbirth, major surgery, severe illness, psychological stress and chemotherapy. The good news is that the abnormal growth behavior associated with telogen effluvium is temporary and reversible.

There are numerous other less common hair loss causes that need to be discounted before a course of treatment is chosen. Traction alopecia is the loss of hair from constant pulling, usually as the result of hair styling. Broken hairs can result in thinning, often caused by excessive styling or exposure to chemicals and sun. Finally, severe illnesses or nutritional deficiencies can cause side effects that may include degrees of hair loss.

I hope this brief e-book has gotten across the message that diagnosing the real causes of hair loss is not always a straightforward process. Once you and your physician have identified a cause, then you can work towards restoring your hair to its former glory. And the good news is, most forms of hair loss can be treated successfully. The next e-book in this series will look at some of the best hair loss treatments currently available.

Sources and Treatment of Hair Loss

On average, people lose about 10% of their hair during a resting phase. Then after about three months, resting hair falls out and new hair begins to grow. The phase of new growing hair typically lasts anywhere from two to six years with hair growing about one-half to one-inch per month. The interesting thing is that as much as 90% of hair on your head is growing at any given time.

Shedding hair is a normal process. In fact, on a normal day, you would lose about 100 hairs although more if you were actually going through significant hair loss. Now, hair loss is usually associated with men but women can also go through hair loss.

The cause of excessive hair loss could be a number of things:

- For starters, if you have undergone major surgery or illness, you might lose more hair for the following three months than you normally do because of stress.
- Another common cause of excessive hair loss is due to hormonal changes within the body. This in itself could be from several things such as having a baby, dealing with an under or overly active thyroid, having estrogen or androgens imbalance, and so on. Then, certain types of drugs can also cause hair loss. In this case, once the medication is stopped, the excessive hair loss usually stops as well.
- The most common culprits include blood thinners, chemotherapy, excessive vitamin A, antidepressants, gout medication, and birth control pills.
- Then, if you have a fungal infection of the scalp, you might also find your hair falling out more than usual. Finally, underlying disease can also be a challenge. For instance, if you are living with something such as diabetes, lupus, or another autoimmune disease, excessive hair loss is common. Remember, by taking the right medication to treat the problem, hair growth generally returns to normal.

Tips!

Although some types of hair loss are genetic, you can also do a few things to help slow down or stop the process. For starters,

- Avoid wearing your hair in cornrows, ponytails, or hot rollers, which tend to pull and stretch hair to the point of breakage.
- In addition, if hair follicles should become inflamed, excessive hair loss may occur. In this case, having your hair permed, colored, or treated with hot oil could be damaging.

The key here is to only, have a professional work on your hair, using professional and safe products.

If the hair loss is extreme and you have tried everything you know from eating healthy to using good hair care products but nothing is working, you might visit with your doctor. First, he or she will look at what is going on with your body to see if medication, infection, or illness could be the problem. If not, **blood work** may be performed to look further at a possible cause. In some cases, your doctor may prescribe certain medication such as hormones for an imbalance or antibiotics for an infection.

Other than that, you will find a number of excellent products now on the market that can help maintain the current amount of hair and in some cases, help with regrowth.

Some superficial follicle infections spontaneously resolve themselves. However, bacterial infections like ***impetigo***, ***furuncles***, ***carbuncles*** and "***hot tub***" ***folliculitis*** may not resolve spontaneously and generally require prescription therapy. All these infections are typically diagnosed by clinical presentation, after which predisposing factors are identified and eliminated.

Fungal folliculitis

As the name suggests fungal folliculitis is caused due to fungal infections. Superficial fungal infections are found in the top layers of the skin; deep fungal infections invade deeper layers of the skin. The infection from hair follicles can also spread to blood or internal organs.

The dermatophytic fungus, *pityrosporum* fungus and the yeast *Candida folliculitis* are the prominent among the fungal folliculitis causes.

Dermatophytic folliculitis is caused most often by a zoophilic species, i.e. fungal species that show attraction to or affinity for animals. The condition presents as follicular pustules around a hardened erythematous (reddened) plaque. A deep fungal penetration causes a high degree of inflammation and determines the extent of hair shaft loss that occurs due to the infection.

Tinea capitis or ringworm of the head is the most important form of pediatric dermatophytic folliculitis. The clinical features of *Tinea capitis* vary considerably depending on the species responsible for the infection. Typically, there is partial alopecia with a varying amount of inflammation.

In the non-inflammatory variants, asymmetrical lesions with short broken hair, 1 to 3 mm in length, are observed. Slight inflammation with scaling may be observed on careful inspection.

The most severe inflammatory reactions are called *kerion* and produce painful boggy masses studded with pustules. These lesions can result in severe hair loss and significant scarring when the disease is in advanced stages. The diagnosis of *Tinea capitis* is established by identifying the organism in infected hairs under the microscope. A diagnosis is often confirmed by cultures.

Tinea barbae is a superficial dermatophytic infection that is limited to the bearded areas of the face and neck and occurs almost exclusively in older adolescent and adult males. The clinical presentation of *Tinea barbae* includes deep folliculitis, red inflammatory papules and pustules with exudation, crusting and associated hair shaft loss. The two main species causing the infection are *T. mentagrophytes* and *T. verrucosum*.

Pityrosporum folliculitis is caused by *pityrosporum* yeasts resulting in an itchy eruption. The lesions are reddish follicular papules and pustules located mainly on the upper back, shoulders and chest.

Candida folliculitis is caused by the Candida species, ubiquitous fungi that most commonly affect humans.

Viral folliculitis

Viral folliculitis involves a variety of viral infections of the hair follicle. Infection by the herpes simple virus (HSV) often progress to form pustular or ulcerated lesions, and eventually a crust. Infection caused by *Molluscum contagiosum* indicates an immuneosuppressed state which manifests as multiple, whitish, itchy papules over the beard area. There are also some reports of folliculitis caused by herpes zoster infection.

Parasitic folliculitis

Parasites causing folliculitis are usually small pathogens that burrow into the hair follicle to live there or lay their eggs. Mites such as *Demodex folliculorum* and *Demodex brevis* are natural hosts of the human pilo-sebaceous follicle.

CHAPTER THREE

DEALING WITH HAIR LOSS

Did I Inherit A Hair Loss Gene?

Keywords: *Hair loss, hair loss remedy, rogaine, thinning hair, bald, balding, women hair, hair, women, pregnant, menopause.*

Summary: *Men who start to go bald even before a mid-life crisis may have their mothers to blame, according to a new study. Researchers have found that the main construction manual for a full head of hair is located on the X chromosome, which sons always inherit from their mothers.*

This genetic storage space contains the so-called androgen receptor gene, a long time balding suspect.

X chromosome and Baldness

Men who start to go bald even before a mid-life crisis may have their mothers to blame, according to a new study. Researchers have found that the main construction manual for a full head of hair is located on the X chromosome, which sons always inherit from their mothers.

This genetic storage space contains the so-called androgen receptor gene, a long time balding suspect. Looking at men who were losing their hair at a relatively young age, a team led by Markus Nothen, PhD, of the ***Life & Brain Center*** at Bonn University, Germany systematically examined all of the genetic patterns within the X chromosome to see why certain hairlines recede faster than others. It's not a pretty picture.

The study, published in the American Journal of Human Genetics, claims that a single alteration in the androgen-receptor gene is the major reason why some men end up going bald before their fathers. Nearly half of bald men would not be bald if they did not have this genetic variation. The hair loss in these younger men, he added, was much more severe than in the men who still had a reason to use a comb in their 60s.

The two approved medicines to treat hair loss (Rogaine and Propecia) need to be taken for a long time to see results. With Propecia, doctors sometimes advise their patients not to expect any results before at least six to eight months. And both need to be used indefinitely to maintain its effect. Once you stop, hair loss will continue.

Although there are only two medicines approved by the Food and Drug Administration (FDA) to treat hair loss, many people are interested in other, alternative treatments. The herb saw palmetto has been used for many years in Europe to treat symptoms of an enlarged prostate and there is some evidence that it may also be effective in treating hair loss.

Dihydrotestosterone (DHT) - The devil in the wood pile

Dihydrotestosterone or DHT as it is known is a very potent hormone in the humane body. This hormone DHT is responsible for giving man his male characteristics when he is just a fetus in his mother's womb. To put things in the simplest of ways, all of us start out in the womb as females, a status decided on by nature. It is during the sixth week of pregnancy that DHT begins to form in the fetus by testosterone, the male hormone, combining with an enzyme called *5 alpha reductase*. It is this DHT that stimulates the growth of the male sex organs and stems the growth of the female genitalia. Now just imaging what would happen if this DHT were to be a scarce commodity during this crucial stage of sex determination in the fetus!

The Anomalies of DHT Deficiency

The result of a deficiency of Dihydrotestosterone in the fetus stage will result in abnormal formation of male sex organs and will produce an infant which will be neither this way nor that, and if the male genitalia are fully formed then there may just be a lack of libido and probably complete sterility.

Let us understand how this happens. Because males with a deficiency of Dihydrotestosterone are born with ambiguous genitalia, this condition is better known as 'Pseudohermaphroditism' the clinical abnormalities of this condition will range from infertility to underdeveloped male with 'Hypospadias' to predominantly developed female external genitalia. The uterus and fallopian tubes in this case are absent because of the normal secretion of the 'müllerian-inhibiting' factor and the testes are intact. Male internal ducts are present but terminate in a blind Pseudovaginal pouch or terminate on the perineum.

How it Works

5-alpha-reductase, the enzyme that converts testosterone to Dihydrotestosterone or DHT, is the cause of this very disturbing disorder. The conversion to DHT involves hydroxylation at the 5 carbon position of the 'A' ring of the steroid molecule. This change flattens the shape of DHT, permitting it to fit perfectly into the androgen receptor in a way that the hormone testosterone cannot. In this way, DHT is bound selectively to the androgen receptors in genital skin and fibroblasts, making its action necessary for the development of normal male genital anatomy in the fetus.

There are therapies available but to what extent they are effective is difficult to say. www.Procerin.com has information on the subject you could use and effective measures to tackle the problem of DHT deficiency as best as present day technology can permit.

Defying Hair Loss at Any Age

Keywords: *Defying Hair Loss at Any Age, defying hair loss, hair transplantation,*

Summary: *Let's face it, hair loss is not a welcome change at any age. With more than 70 percent of men experiencing male pattern baldness at some point in their lives, many of them seek a remedy.*

Aging and Hair Loss

Let's face it, hair loss is not a welcome change at any age. With more than 70 percent of men experiencing male pattern baldness at some point in their lives, many of them seek a remedy.

Hair loss treatments come in many varieties, but only a few work. Possibly the most reliable and permanent solution to this problem is hair transplantation - a minor surgical procedure done under local anesthesia.

Regardless of a man's age or amount of baldness, the latest techniques in hair transplantation can provide what hair loss sufferers want the most - a confident, more youthful appearance.

Bill Wellington, an 83-year-old retired CIA economist and Army Air Force Pilot originally from Detroit, first started noticing his hair loss at 14 or 15. In college, he secretly studied hair loss on his own and even talked to a hair consultant, hoping to find a remedy. Despite these attempts, he continued to lose his hair.

One college hockey teammate remarked that Wellington refused to wet his hair in the shower for fear of losing it.

"I always carried that element of personal insecurity that surfaced when I prepared for work or showered after hockey. It was the receding hair line," Wellington said.

When he fought in World War II, he used his helmet and cap to conceal his problem, but it stayed on his mind. Years later, after he left the Army and had a successful career and a loving family, his hair loss continued to bother him.

The biggest problem, he says, was his loss of self-confidence which stemmed from his baldness. For instance, while taking a family photo, his children commented, "Hey Dad, you're really getting bald."

"The old comic reply, 'hair today, gone tomorrow' got a chuckle but did little to bolster my ego," Wellington said.

After attending a free seminar on hair transplantation, he decided to get treatment from the doctors at Elliott & True, a medical practice specializing in hair transplantation, and he has been satisfied ever since. He still plays organized hockey for a Maryland seniors team called the *Geri-Hatricks*, which he named. He says younger players always compliment his healthy-looking hair.

At the office of doctors Robert H. True and Robert J. Dorin, patients from 25 to 80 get their own natural, growing hair back thanks to the latest hair transplant technology.

"The results are quite impressive nowadays, and they seem to have the same positive effect on a patient's well-being, regardless of his age," True said.

Develop a Strategy for Dealing with Premature Hair Loss

Keywords: Hair loss, baldness, alopecia

Abstract: This e-book outlines the factors you need to consider in developing a strategy for hair regrowth.

What you need to identify the Best Hair Loss Treatments

The fact you are reading this probably indicates you have concerns about the rate of your hair loss. Baldness may sometimes be a source of amusement to those with a full head of hair, but premature hair loss at any age can be the cause of intense concern to those affected.

But you can do something about this! By following the guidelines suggested in this e-book you will place yourself in a position to identify a hair loss treatment that not only works but also fits in with your lifestyle and preferences.

To achieve this you must truthfully answer four simple questions:

1. What is the true cause of your hair loss?

   Most instances of hair loss in men, for example, can be attributed to androgenetic alopecia (male pattern baldness) but you must be certain as this will influence your choice of hair loss treatment. To be completely certain you should consult with your physician.

2. How far has your hair loss progressed?

   It is crucial to realize that the sooner you start treating hair loss, the greater your chances of success. You need to identify the pattern of hair loss as this will help establish both the cause and most effective treatment option.

3. What hair loss treatment options are you prepared to consider?

   Your answer to this question will depend on a number of factors including the type and extent of hair loss, what treatments have been tried previously, your personal preferences with regard to using medications or natural remedies and the amount you are prepared to spend.

4. Do you have sufficient patience and determination to succeed?

   There really are no miracle cures for premature hair loss. Equally, there are treatments that can halt and even reverse this condition, but none of them will work overnight. Treatments take time to work and there is no such thing as a remedy that suits everyone.

When you have given proper consideration to these questions you will find yourself in a better position to choose the hair loss treatment that best suits your circumstances. It you're still not sure, talk to your physician or carry out more research. But you need to be clear on one point - the longer you delay, the more difficult your path to hair regrowth will be.

Don't Lose Hair

Keywords: *Hair loss,*

Abstract: Men and hair loss seems always to have been a losing combination. Although male pattern hair loss is very common—two out of three men will experience it—and is hardly ever associated with serious health risks, it's hard to imagine a common condition that is met with more anxiety.

Male Pattern Hair Loss

Men and hair loss seems always to have been a losing combination. Although male pattern hair loss is very common—two out of three men will experience it—and is hardly ever associated with serious health risks, it's hard to imagine a common condition that is met with more anxiety. But much of the stigma surrounding male hair loss is due to half-truths and exaggerations. So if you start noticing there's not as much hair up there, don't pull out the rest of it in worry—take our quiz below and learn what's going on with your body and how you can slow the follicle fallout.

If you're losing hair, it's male pattern baldness.

False. It's true that for 95 percent of men who lose their hair, male pattern baldness, or androgenetic alopecia, is the culprit. With this condition, an enzyme called *5-alpha reductase* converts testosterone to dihydrotestosterone, a hormone that causes hair follicles to shut down hair production. Male pattern baldness can begin appearing in men in their 20s and usually progresses slowly from the front or apex of the scalp, or both.

But male pattern baldness is not the only cause of male hair loss—and it's important to talk to your physician or dermatologist to determine the cause, because it can point to certain health problems. For example,

- If your hair is falling out quickly and in small patches, it may be a sign of alopecia areata, an autoimmune disease in which the body attacks the hair.
- Stress can also lead to rapid hair loss. In these cases, the hair usually regrows after several months.

- Other causes include a severe ailment or major surgery; protein, vitamin B, or iron deficiencies; medication complications; or thyroid disease.

It's your mother's fault.

False. Male pattern baldness is a largely genetic characteristic that can be inherited from either your mother or your father. It's even possible to acquire the hair-loss gene from both parents. In fact, the same gene also causes hair loss in women, although because of hormonal differences, women tend to lose their hair in small amounts all over their scalp.

There's hope.

True. Here's the good news: In many cases, male pattern baldness can be treated. In the early stages, many conventional physicians prescribe either *Minoxidil* lotion, applied topically, or *Finasteride*, taken orally. These medications have been shown to slow hair loss in many patients and, in some cases, cause hair to grow back. According to Robert Brodell, MD, professor of internal medicine in the dermatology section at Northeastern Ohio Universities College of Medicine, complications associated with both drugs are minimal, but there are downsides. Not only are the medications expensive, but they only work for as long as you take them. "I tell my patients that they are going to be on one of those medicines for 5 years or 10 years or 15 years, until they are married and have kids and don't care anymore," says Brodell. "And then when they stop their medicine, we fully expect them to start losing their hair again." Great strides are being made in the field of hair transplants, but like any invasive therapy, these procedures are expensive and time-consuming and should not be undertaken lightly.

If surgery or drug therapies aren't for you, a number of naturopathic remedies might offer similar results—without the high cost. Keith F. Zeitlin, ND, a naturopathic physician with a private practice in Connecticut, recommends the herbs saw palmetto (*Serenoa repens*) and stinging nettle root (*Urtica dioica*), and the supplement beta-sitosterol, which all appear to work similarly to conventional medicines by shutting down the enzyme 5-alpha reductase's creation of dihydrotestosterone, the hormone that ceases hair production. "If we can inhibit that enzyme, we can actually inhibit hair loss," says Zeitlin. (For more information, see "Herbs and Supplements for Hair Loss," below.)

Another option is mesotherapy, a treatment in which very short needles are used to inject homeopathic remedies; vitamins such as biotin; or conventional medicines such as minoxidil just underneath the surface of the scalp. "The skin is used as a natural time-release system," says practitioner Harry Adelson, ND, a Utah-based pain-medicine specialist. "Whatever it is you are injecting remains in the area for up to a week and continually penetrates down into the deeper tissue."

You can live a hair-healthy lifestyle.

True. Although there's no apparent validity to the old wives' tales that sexual activity or excessive hat wearing can cause hair loss, other lifestyle choices may indeed hurt your hair. In fact, it might make more sense to keep that hat on; a study conducted at the University Hospital of Zurich in Switzerland proposed that ultraviolet rays from the sun might injure hair follicles (Dermatology, 2003, vol. 207, no. 4). How you clean and care for your hair may also be a factor in hair loss. According to the American Academy of Dermatology, too many chemical treatments such as dying, straightening, and bleaching, as well as excessive washing, towel drying, and brushing, may weaken or damage your hair, causing it to break or fall out.

Those worried about hair loss should also reevaluate their diets. Zeitlin warns that very large doses of vitamin A can lead to vitamin A toxicity and eventual hair loss. He recommends his patients replace vitamin A-rich foods and saturated fats, which may also encourage hair loss, with green vegetables, whole grains, essential fatty acids, and other foods rich in hair-healthy vitamins and minerals such as zinc. What you drink may also play a role: According to a 2003 study, alcohol consumption may aggravate hair loss (British Journal of Dermatology, 2003, vol. 149, no. 6).

Hair loss is a bad thing.

False. Let's not forget the cheapest, easiest, and safest treatment for male pattern hair loss: doing nothing at all. After all, hair loss is not usually a health concern and, despite what our culture may sometimes suggest, there's nothing wrong with showing a little skin—on your head, that is. After all, look at Patrick Stewart, Bruce Willis, and Sean Connery. "I certainly wouldn't recommend that anybody have their male pattern baldness treated who isn't bothered by it," says Brodell. "I'm losing my hair, and I'm not using any of these treatments."

CHAPTER FOUR

HAIR LOSS REMEDY

Do Natural Hair Loss Remedies Have Any Real Relevance?

Abstract: *Natural remedies, Hair loss remedies, natural hair loss remedies,*

Summary*: This e-book examines whether natural hair loss treatments have anything tangible to offer today.*

Do Natural Hair Loss Remedy Work?

The effectiveness of modern hair loss treatments is clear for all to see, but many people simply prefer not to use strong chemicals or non-natural substances.

If you fall into this category, does this mean you'll just have to accept an ever-decreasing head of hair? The answer to this is an unequivocal NO!

Many natural hair loss remedies, both traditional and contemporary, have shown their worth in reducing and reversing hair loss. They are also perceived as being free from side effects and even deliver additional health benefits.

Why then, don't we hear a lot more about these natural hair loss remedies? Simply because claims of cures cannot be made without FDA approval, and obtaining the FDA seal of approval involves lengthy and expensive scientific research that only major companies can afford. Even the biggest companies could not recoup the costs of such a process as no-one can control the rights to common natural substances such as basic foods and vitamins.

The big question however is, do natural hair loss remedies work? Firstly, hair growth at root level is a living part of the body that depends on sound nutrition, just like any other part of the body. The importance of vitamins, minerals and other nutritional elements in maintaining healthy hair cannot be disputed.

Secondly, the role of herbs and plants in treating numerous ailments is receiving increased recognition after years of neglect, and hair loss is no exception. Many herbal remedies for both internal and external use are offering new hope to people suffering from premature hair loss.

Thirdly, traditional hair loss remedies may still have something to offer. Ancient literature and folklore reveal that our ancestors went to great lengths to treat thinning hair. Some of the more acceptable traditional approaches are now being incorporated into many potential treatment regimes.

Choosing Hair Loss Remedy

Keywords: hair loss cures, hair loss solutions, herbal hair loss solutions, hair care remedy.

Abstract: Hair loss solutions have become a craze in the modern world. However, one must be careful while choosing a hair care remedy. The herbal hair loss solutions are good choices as they have no side effect and are very effective as well.

Hair Loss Remedy

Your external appearance and beauty of your hair contributes a lot to your personality. It is for this simple reason that there is too much rush for buying the cosmetic products The market today is flooded with a variety of cosmetic products which offer all kind s of hair loss solutions and hair loss cures.

Be careful while choosing a hair loss remedy

But before you choose a hair loss remedy for you, beware of the fake hair loss solutions and hair loss cures. It is always better to consult a doctor if you are suffering from hair loss. Hair loss can take place due to various medical conditions. It is quite possible that your hair loss problem is not of a permanent nature and could be cured by some simple treatments.

Do not let over-the-counter drugs dupe you. You must diagnose the actual cause of your problem and search for the right kind of remedy.

Herbal hair loss remedies

Herbal hair loss solutions play important role in countering hair problems. Herbal remedies have always been popular in traditional Indian and Chinese medications. Of late, they have been dominating the Western world as well.

Reasons for their popularity

There are mainly two reasons for their popularity.

First, they have fewer side effects. They are the ideal hair loss cures if you are looking for safe, risk free procedures.

Secondly, they are very effective. No, they do not stand for any overnight solution. But you may certainly notice a difference in the thickness, strength, volume and sheen in your hair after using a herbal hair loss remedy. Herbal remedies

- Increase circulation
- Disinfect the scalp and
- Stimulate hair growth.

There are some herbal remedies which also block the synthesis of DHT (dihydrotestosterone) the natural inhibitor of hair growth.

Some of the herbal hair loss cures that you may find useful are as follows

- **Green tea** (*Camellia sinesis*) - Catechins in green tea inhibit the enzyme **5-alpha-reductase** that converts testosterone into hair-unfriendly DHT. Therefore drinking green tea everyday is a fruitful treatment for male pattern baldness.

- **Ayurvedic Antistress Tea** – Consuming this mixed drink of Nardostachys jatamamsi and Bacopa monnieri 2 to 3 times a day relieves stress and prevents hair loss.

- **Ginko biloba** - It intensifies blood circulation to the scalp and skin. Consuming 120-160mg of dry Ginko extract every day can keep your hair follicles rejuvenated.

- **Saw palmetto** (*Seranoa repens*) – This herb is known for slowing hair loss and encouraging hair regrowth. It is a core element of many hair loss formulations. The recommended dose is a 160mg capsule twice each day.

- **He Shou Wu** (*Polygonum multiflorum*) - This Chinese herb is used in many commercial preparations for hair loss remedy.

- **Pygeum** (*Pygeum africanum*) - Used to treat prostate problems and male pattern baldness. Recommended dosage is 60-500mg per day.

- **Stinging Nettle** (*Urtica diocia*) - It blocks the conversion of testosterone into DHT. It delivers wonderful results if taken in combination with Pygeum and Saw Palmetto.

If you are choosing a cosmetic hair product for yourself, read its label carefully. Choose a product that is based on the above herbal supplements or contain the natural hair care products.

Besides these herbal remedies there are various dietary supplements which are essential for supplying the adequate nutrition to the hair follicles and ensure good health to your hair. Eating a diet rich in vitamin, minerals, and protein is the best hair loss remedy one can choose.

Dynamic Pattern Hair Loss Discovery. Treatment and Recovery through Scalp Hygiene "Healthy Scalps Grow Healthy Hair"

Keywords: *Hair loss, hair loss treatments, male pattern hair loss, female pattern hair loss, hair loss recovery, hair restoration, scalp conditions, hair loss treatments, hair loss heredity, hair loss treatment products*

Summary: *Finally, the essential step and logical solution for naturally treating pattern hair loss and problem scalp conditions has been discovered. No surgery, grafts or gimics, just scalp health. Owner of Scalp & Skin Works, Scalp Clinic and Salon, Karen Crever announces the creation of System Scalp & Skin, a cleansing alternative dedicated to pattern hair loss recovery, providing logical, natural solutions for hair loss and problematic scalp conditions. The industry of scalp health recovery is born.*

Hair loss affects approximately 50 million men and women in the United States, but few people understand how and why they are losing their hair. Although genetic dispositions contribute, it's primarily the lack of epidermal health that suppresses normal hair and skin production. Throughout Karen's 25 year career, clients complained of itchy scalp conditions and pattern hair loss. There had to be natural, non-invasive treatment alternatives to hydro cortisone creams, hair grafts and hair transplant surgery. Hair loss treatment products, weaves and supplements have shown little or no results. She was determined to find a solution.

Karen had an extraordinary epiphany. Why no one had considered the obvious reason of poor scalp health as the underlying cause is anyone's guess. She discovered pattern hair loss involved more than just heredity. **Scalp & Skin Works** has revealed the crucial step and logical solution for pattern hair loss and undesirable scalp conditions. The problem. Pattern hair loss is multifaceted and more complicated than she, and obviously everyone else realized. The abundance and over production of excess skin layers, perspiration and impurities like sticky sebum clogs, and follicle parasites all contribute to hair loss.

The solution. Recovery begins, by detoxifying the scalp, restoring proper hygiene and fostering healthy environments conducive for normal scalp and skin growth. "Clients are able to actually see their scalp condition, and watch the removal of impurities with the assistance of a cosmetic microscope and monitor as the clinician works. It's an interactive process. Most are amazed and fascinated at what they see, eyes glues to the screen. Others get grossed out and just don't look". Customers are very pleased with their results. "I had given up. I had tried other hair loss treatments and did not want to do transplant surgery. Then *System Scalp & Skin* showed me that I could re-grow my own hair through their scalp hygiene process. It wasn't long and I could actually see new hair growing in. My hair is now getting thicker and my "halo" is shrinking. *System Scalp & Skin* works!" Kevin Buchan, Oil Industry Lobbyist, Cameron Park CA.

A Hair Loss Cure for Men

Procerin

Procerin as a natural remedy for hair loss has been found to be effective in reversing hair loss in men caused by *Androgenetic alopecia;* the most common cause of male hair loss. Thinning hair and receding hairlines are often referred to as widow's peak. Basically, men suffering from *Androgenetic alopecia* have extremely high levels of the chemical dihydrotestosterone (DHT), a by-product of the major male hormone *testosterone*. When this hormone is converted into DHT, the results are hair loss and this is where Procerin steps in and blocks the production of DHT and unlike other medications does not react with *testosterone*.

Procerin has been scientifically designed to help men retain and regrow their hair. The 17 active ingredients are all natural and herbal, containing vitamins, minerals and DHT inhibitors. The ingredients include but not limited to:

- Saw Palmetto Berries
- Gotu Kola
- Nettles
- Magnesium
- Zinc Sulfate
- Siberian Ginseng
- Vitamin B-6
- Pumpkin Seed Meal
- CJ-11 Factor
- CJ-9 Factor
- Mura Puma Root

Because the *Procerin* hair loss treatment product for men contains only natural ingredients the only known side effect is mild stomach discomfort for the first few days. If you are suffering an illness it is wise to consult your doctor before use, especially if you are currently taking a MAOI inhibitor.

Studies have shown that *Procerin* is more effective as a natural hair loss remedy in men aged between 18-35 and those whose hair is still in a growth phase. Men that still have growing hair experience an increase in hair count, and improvement in both hairline and thinning at the crown of their head, because hair grows at an extremely slow rate (about 1" every two months). It's best to take *Procerin* for at least 1-2 months before results can be expected, but some users of *Procerin* have reported good results after only 2 weeks. Most men take 1-3 months before significant increases in hair count occur, not bad when compared to *Propecia* that can take up to 6 months for good hair growth results.

So, does Procerin work?

Procerin has had many good results with many success stories and the companies boast that *Procerin;* the natural hair loss remedy works with 92% of men who suffer *Androgenetic alopecia* the most common cause of hair. *Procerin* is a cost effective alternative to other hair loss treatment products like *Propecia & Rogaine* and unlike prescription medication, *Procerin* is backed by a 90-Day Unconditional, No questions asked, Money Back Guarantee so you have nothing to lose except to gain your hair of course.

Renew

Hair loss on account of any specific reason like medication, abnormal hormone levels or infection of scalp can be treated. The most troublesome and the most common forms of baldness is the common male/female baldness in which the hair recedes along the temples and the forehead in the case of men and recedes in density all over in the case of women. Such baldness is usually genetic. Genetic baldness is usually caused by an enzyme *Alpha reductase* that converts testosterone to DHT. DHT leads to the shrinking of hair follicles. This results in the generation of thinner and weaker strands of hair that fall off very quickly.

The special herbal hair care product *Renew* contains a group of herbs that provide overall scalp and hair root nutrition and also help in the control of dandruff. The special herbs in *Renew* help in stopping hair follicle shrinkage. Regular use leads to reversal of shrinkage and promotes hair gain. *Renew* is helpful in all kinds of hair loss situations.

Renew is available in the form of hair oil that has to be applied loc ally. Local application means that unlike when systemic hair loss medicines like *Fenasteride* and *Dutasteride,* hair growth does not happen in undesirable areas like the back or the bums.

Massaging of hair and scalp with *Renew* provides additional nutrition to the scalp and prevents hair loss. Massaging also increases the blood circulation in the scalp and this keeps the hair roots strong.

Direction for use

Part your hair and apply *Renew* all over the scalp, massage the scalp gently with fingers in a circular motion so that the oil gets absorbed into the scalp. Leave for an hour and then wash with mild shampoo if required. Alternatively, you could apply Renew to your hair and scalp before going to sleep and then wash your hair in the morning.

Side Effects

Renew has no known side effects.

Composition

Each 10 ml of *Renew* oil contains:

Eclipta alba 3%

Herpestis/Bacopa monnieria 2%

Emblica officinalis 2%

Cyperus scariosus 1%

Vetiveria zizanioides 1%

Santalum album 1%

Pongamia glabra 1%

Crataeva nurvala 0.5%

Abrus precatorius 0.5%

Glycyrrhiza glabra 0.5%

Nardostachys jatamansi 0.5%

Valeriana jatamansi 0.5%

More information about this and other health products at: http://www.healthstore.4yz.com

And see this and other products in http://www.allthemarket.net

Discover How to Stop Hair Loss - Grow More Hair

Keywords: *Hair loss, hair thinning, hair baldness*

Abstract: *Hair loss and hair thinning occurs because not enough hair nutrients reach the hair roots. Here are some natural remedies that you can use to increase the blood circulation to your scalp to keep the hair you have or to stop hair thinning.*

Factors Responsible for Hair Loss and Baldness

In one of my other e-books, I revealed that plugged hair follicles are one of the main conditions that start hair thinning and baldness. The other condition is insufficient blood circulation in the scalp.

When you don't have enough blood circulating in your scalp, then your hair roots don't get enough nutrients to support the life and strength of your hair in the follicle.

The hardest place to get good circulation is at the top of your scalp. It is the furthest point away from your heart. It is the area that is less stimulated. The sides of your head are stimulated as you sleep and move your head around the pillow. That is one reason why most people still have hair on the sides of their head while the top is completely bald.

So what are the ways you can increase blood circulation to the top of your head?

Here are two ways to do it:

- Use herbal remedies to increase body and scalp blood circulation
- Use hot and cold hydrotherapy

Use herbal remedies to increase body and scalp blood circulation

There are several herbs that provide increase circulation to all parts of the body. Two good standby remedies are *ginkgo biloba* and *Cayenne pepper*. Use ginkgo biloba as indicated on the label. Ginkgo increases the blood circulation in the brain and all parts of the head.

Use Cayenne pepper in the formulation made by **Heart Foods Company**. This Cayenne strengthens the heart giving it the ability to pump blood to the furthest reaches of the body.

There are two other herbal formulations that have recently come out to provide increase circulation to all parts of the body - **Vital** *cell* and *Arjuna*.

Vital cell is a Chinese herbal combination that is available in the US. It is a powerful remedy that helps to re-establish small veins that have closed off. This creates more pathways for blood to go where it is needed and where it once went.

Arjuna is another herb that comes from another country - India. It is now readily available in the US. Arjuna is the latest herb to be exposed as good for preventing and reducing arthrosclerosis. By reducing narrowing of the arteries in the head, strokes can be avoided and a side benefit is the scalp get more blood.

Use Hot and Cold Hydrotherapy

I have talked about this natural way of bringing more blood into the scalp. It's a technique I use every time I shower. At the end of your shower, run hot water over your head for 20 seconds, turn the hot water off and allow the cold water to run over your head for 20 seconds.

Do this hot-cold water technique three - four times and end with the cold water. This technique allow blood to move in and out of the lower layers of your scalp giving you a blood massage and providing more nutrients to your hair roots. As a side benefit, you are bringing in more blood to your brain giving you more brain power as long as use this technique.

Use herbs to improve you blood circulation to your scalp and use hot-cold water to blood massage your scalp. By doing this, you will find less hair loss and you may even start to see some hair growth.

Easy Hair Loss Cure

Keywords: *Easy hair loss cure, hair problems, hair loss treatment, hair loss treatment products, hair loss, hair, hair loss solutions, hair care, hair loss remedy.*

Summary: *The e-book 'Easy Hair Loss Cure' is of great help to you if you are suffering with hair problems. After reading this e-book you will be agree with the fact that 'cure of hair problems is easy' and hair problems is like any other problems, which can be solved easily and effectively.*

Simple Hair Loss Care

Hair loss and baldness is a common problem in our society. A number of men and women are facing hair loss problems and seeking help. Hair problem badly affects one's social activities and especially the women. About 90% of men and women are suffering hair problems, sometime it is thinning of hair, sometime it is falling of hair and some time it is becoming bald.

In general, a person with less hair on his / her head is considered as less smart / beautiful as his / her counterpart who has hairy head with healthy hair. Hair loss is clinically diagnosed as the deficiency of Biotin which is a water-soluble B-vitamin. It's part of the B complex group of vitamins. Vitamin B7 and vitamin H are other synonyms of Biotin.

It is said that, 'prevention is better than cure', so a person need to take vitamin H rich diet to maintain his / her body and hair health, as biotin is also important for other bodily functions. But no problem comes calling in life, so if you are having hair problems, then you need to take necessary steps to prevent further loss and ultimately baldness.

Now, you definitely will be interested in knowing the steps one must take in the case of Hair Problems.

Here is little 'Easy Hair Loss Cure' advice, which you will like to follow, if you are facing Hair Loss Problems.

Different types of lotions, various medicines and shampoos in different fragrances are available in the market stores to protect your hair. You can buy these hair loss treatment products from a medical store in your locality. There are products, which you can buy only after a physician's prescription. The choice of selecting a hair loss treatment product totally depends on the level of suffering you are going through.

The clinical root cause of hair loss may be any, like hereditary, hormonal imbalance and aging etc. And hence an individual need to receive medications accordingly. The blocking of hair follicles is found to be one major condition for hair problems. A hormone called dihydrotestosterone in excessive quantity does the blocking of hair follicles, which ultimately results into hair problems. Dihydrotestosterone is also pronounced as DHT. The effect of DHT in hair follicles can be neutralized using 5 – alpha reductase, which is an inhibitor.

Nugen HP, Revivogen, and *Hair Genesis* are some of the common hair loss treatment products available in pharmacies and drug stores. All these medicines help in reducing the level of DHT and thus help in the control of hair loss and promote healthy hair.

Nugen HP controls your problems naturally. This blocks the DHT in follicles and thus cures your hair problems. If you are facing hair problems, you must have to take proper nutritious balanced diet. Take a diet full with proteins, vitamins and minerals.

Hair genesis is very effective in hair problems. It is a natural DHT blocker and prevents hair loss in males. Many more products are available in the medical and pharmacy stores, but while using any product, taking diet rich in nutrition is also equally important.

You also can use hair conditioners to prevent hair loss. *Revivogen, Folligen, Tricomin*, and *Nisim* are some of the hair conditioners.

Minoxdil is a drug, which is effective in the case of youngsters' hair problems. So, no matter if you are facing hair problems, a number of drugs, and conditioners are there to help you prevent hair loss. But be cautious, take the advice of your doctor and have food enriched with vitamins and minerals and proteins. Hair loss is curable and with little extra effort you can have healthy hair on your head.

CHAPTER FIVE

BALDNESS-GOOD OR BAD

BALDNESS

Keywords: Bald, Bald Heads, Bald Women, Bald Men

Abstract: Over the ages, baldness has been considered a disease. Lately, it has also been followed as a fashion. However, greater numbers of people still feel that a head covered by hair is always more attractive than a bald one.

The Effect of Follicle Shrinkage

Over the ages, baldness has been considered a disease. Lately, it has also been followed as a fashion. However, greater numbers of people still feel that a head covered by hair is always more attractive than a bald one.

Every month, hair grows by about 1 inch. Normally, around 85% of the hair on your head is always in the growing phase at any time, and 15% is not. Five years is the maximum amount of time for which hair normally lives. Considering these statistics, it is difficult to understand the causes of hair loss, which might be more apparent in a few of us.

The follicle is a cavity in the skin where the hair sits. In cases of hair loss this follicle shrinks over time, thereby causing shorter and thinner hair. The final result could be a very tiny follicle with no hair in it. Usually the hair grows back, but for people who are already balding, the follicle is unable to grow a new hair.

Peladic is a disease which leads to hair loss. Some people are repelled at the sight of a bald head, and fear going bald themselves. This fear is called *peladophobia*.

In the dating arena, some women feel very strongly against men with bald heads, and insist that dating a bald guy is almost next to impossible. However, many women do not mind dating a man with a purposely shaved head. It's almost like dating on the basis of your capability to grow more hair on your head.

Balding Solution for Men and Women

Keywords: *Male baldness, female baldness, DHT, androgenetic alopecia*

Abstract: *Both men and women, are genetically pre-disposed to produce more DHT than the normal individuals. It is this accumulation of DHT and its effect on the cells inside the hair follicle and root which is one of the primary causes of male and female pattern balding.*

Factors Responsible for Male and Female Baldness

Androgenetic alopecia (male and female pattern balding) is by far the most common cause of hair loss amongst men and a serious problem for many women. There are three important components which are responsible for both female and male balding:

1. A genetic predisposition for balding to occur.

2. Excessive presence of male hormones.

3. Aging - enough time for the first two factors to occur.

Both men and women produce male hormones that have a useful role to play in both sexes; but the fact that *androgens* occur in much higher concentrations in men explains why male pattern baldness is more common than the female balding.

DHT THE ROOT CAUSE OF HAIR LOSS

It is the metabolism of male hormones (androgen/testosterone) that is the main cause of hair loss and male and female pattern balding in both men and women.

The metabolism of *androgen* involves an enzyme called **5 alpha reductase** which combines with the hormone (testosterone) and converts it to DHT (di-hydro-testosterone). DHT is a natural metabolite of our body.

The cause of male and female pattern balding

Some individuals, both men and women, are genetically pre-disposed to produce more DHT than the normal individuals. It is this accumulation of DHT and its effect on the cells inside the hair follicle and root which is one of the primary causes of male and female pattern balding.

When DHT gets into the hair follicle and root, especially a region called the **dermal papilla**, it changes the cell' activity and prevents necessary proteins, vitamins and minerals from providing nourishment needed to sustain life in the hairs of those follicles. Consequently, hair follicles are reproduced at a much slower rate. This shortens their growing stage (*anagen phase*) and or lengthens their resting stage (*telogen phase*) of the follicle.

DHT also causes hair follicle to shrink and get progressively smaller and finer. This process is known as **miniaturization** and causes the hair to ultimately fall. DHT induced *androgenetic aloepcia* is responsible for 95% of all hair loss.

Blocking the synthesis of DHT at the molecular level forms the basis for the treatment of MPHL (male pattern hair loss) and FPHL (female pattern hair loss). There are many natural DHT blockers and a number of drugs which are used for medical hair restoration.

Baldness Solutions to End the Hair-raising Story of Hair Loss

Hair is a striking feature of human body. Hair loss, especially by female/male pattern baldness is a matter of great concern. Pattern baldness is particularly a very troubling condition. In this type of baldness the hair is regularly lost at both the temples and top of the skull. At last the person is left with a horseshoe pattern in the head.

Male pattern baldness (*androgenetic alopecia*) is the chief devil that causes hair loss. With age, one suffers from this disorder by acquiring the genetic predisposition and presence of male hormones. Contrary to the common perception, hereditary baldness is not a must in each generation. However, if one's father is completely bald and one loses hair at an early stage, then he is said to be in male pattern baldness due to alopecia and 95% of complete baldness occurs by alopecia.

Excess amount of male hormone also causes hair loss. Besides, stress, improper nutrition and pollution together accelerate the baldness. One under stress will loss hair at double the speed of a normal human.

NOTE: Taking dietary supplement and/or external application of cosmetics is fruitless to stop baldness.

Fortunately, there are several baldness solutions, the most popular ones being hair transplantation surgery, scalp reduction surgery and scalp flap surgery.

1. **Hair Transplant Surgery--**there is no such thing as true hair transplant. Surgeons replace the bald area with some other hair-healthy area of the head. Hence, the name hair replacement transplant. Hair transplant works when there is enough donor hairs. Victims of female/male pattern balding are the best candidates for hair transplant. If you still have hair growing anywhere around the scalp flaps, hair transplantation can be easy and effective.

2. **Scalp Reduction Surgery--**is a popular balding solution to cure the baldness caused by flaking scalps. It can be done in conjunction with hair transplants and involves surgically removing of a portion of the balding area, which causes the bald spot to be smaller. This means that there are fewer areas to graft to the head during a hair transplant.

3. **Scalp Flap Surgery--**is an invasive procedure that involves surgically removing a portion of healthy scalp and hair from the back or sides of the head and transplanting it on the bald areas. This creates a new hairline for the males who suffer from male pattern baldness. Scalp flaps are usually performed on patients who have complete balding in the front area of the scalp. Those candidates whose hair is just beginning to thin or is thinning in patches in random areas spanning the head may want to choose a different type of treatment.

Can Female Hair Loss Make Me Totally Bald?

Keywords: Hair thinning, hair loss, hair, hair growth, fast hair growth, bald, balding, female hair loss, menopause.

Abstract: View the pattern that affects women only. Loss of female hair is not the same as male hair loss determined by heredity. Female hair loss is temporary and is seldom an advance warning of baldness. Transient loss of hair should not, however, be ignored. It is possible for a woman to suffer from hormonal hair loss leading to baldness.

Some of the most common causes are:

1. Pregnancy
2. Severe emotional stress
3. Under medical treatment
4. Hormonal hair loss

Is there a relationship between hair loss and menopause?

The most common cause of hair loss is low thyroid function, which is common among menopausal women. Other causes include, but are not limited to:

- changes in hormone levels,
- increased testosterone,
- increased stress, which can either be physical stress, or emotional stress,
- various medications, scalp/dermatological issues and
- Heredity.

Any time sudden hair loss is experienced, one must consider events which took place up to three months prior to the hair loss, as factors affecting hair loss can often take up to three months to have an effect, i.e. were you diagnosed with something new in the past few months? Did you start taking medication during the past few months? Did you go through a traumatic experience? Subsequently, any treatments for hair loss should be given at least three months to have noticeable effects.

There are of course various ways to solve hair problems, such as:

- Wig / toupe
- Hair-weaving (weaving in extra hair)
- Hair transplant
- Cosmetic hair treatment courses
- Therapy

There are only a few products available worldwide which have been conclusively proven to combat hair loss. They are *Aminexil*, *Alopesan 400*, *Maxilène*, *Minoxidil* and *Finasteride*. It's very important for you as a consumer to know this if you are thinking of taking steps to combat your hair loss. *Rogaine* is another one of the more popular brand names in the hair loss treatment industry.

Cure your Baldness & Alopecia the Natural Way (Chinese Herbs)

Keywords: Balding, baldness, thinning, losing hair, alopecia cure treatment.

Abstract: An expert information on the best natural methods in which to cure alopecia to prevent thinning hair & baldness

Treatment for Baldness and Alopecia

A recent media broadcast on UK television as part of an experiment to cure alopecia and treat thinning hair and baldness uncovered the beneficial factors of using Chinese herbs in treating alopecia.

There are a number of Chinese herbs that can be beneficial for this condition. Chinese medicine treats the root imbalances in the body that result in alopecia. When the body is brought into balance, symptoms resolve themselves and slowly disappear.

The first is a pattern of Liver and Kidney Deficiency. This means that the energy of the body that normally nourishes the hair follicles is deficient. When herbs are used to nourish the Liver and Kidney, hair can start to grow back. The second pattern is toxic heat in the body. This means that there is an inflammatory condition in the body that is a result of excess acidity from a poor diet, exposure to pollution or other toxins, or an infection. In most people with alopecia areata, these two conditions exist in combination with each other.

It is necessary to reduce inflammation and acidity in the body while nourishing the cooling yin energy of the body that nourishes hair growth.

He Shou Wu, Polygonum otherwise known as *Fo-ti*, is one herb that can be beneficial for people with *alopecia areata*.

This herb has been used traditionally in China for graying hair and premature hair loss. It is a general tonic for the brain and the body, and can improve the quality of hair growth on the head. It can take three to six months of use to see the full benefits of *Fo-ti*. The Chinese have also traditionally used this herb as a longevity tonic.

Ligustrum and *eclipta* are also two Chinese herbs used to nourish hair growth by strengthening the Liver and Kidney Yin energy of the body. Research done in China have shown that these herbs can promote hair growth in people with *alopecia areata*.

Chinese wolfberries are also a general body tonic that improve blood circulation to hair follicles of the head. This herb can work well in combination with the herbs listed above.

In order to clear the inflammation and acidity that can trigger alopecia, mint, dandelion, and honeysuckle herbs can be used in combination.

Some supplements that may be of benefit in combination with Chinese herbs include vitamin C, flaxseed oil, and nettle tea. All of these are anti-inflammatory and detoxifying to the body. Eating black beans and black sesame seeds can also be helpful when taken alongside Chinese herbs.

Chinese herbs are a safe, natural, effective, health-promoting way to treat *alopecia areata* and increase hair growth.

In my next e-book I will write about another natural cure for Alopecia that has been found to be beneficial in treating thinning hair & baldness. If you want to no more about how to treat and cure alopecia, visit my sites listed below http://www.allthemarket.net

A Guide to Balding Men's Hairstyle

Keywords: *Baldness, Balding hairstyles, balding men hairstyles, comb over, shaved head*

Abstract: *Are you frustrated trying to find information on the internet about balding men's hairstyles? Read this section for a lighthearted but informative guide to balding hairstyles.*

In Search of the Perfect Balding Hairstyle

It's unbelievable how difficult it is to find any decent information on the internet about balding men's hairstyles.

You'll know this yourself if you've ever tried to do a search on Google for 'balding men's hairstyles', 'hairstyles for balding men', 'balding hairstyles' or any other amount of variations on the theme.

This is surprising considering how many balding men there are who deserve a decent hairstyle as much as anyone else…

So… faced with this injustice I've put together my own guide to balding men's hairstyles…

It's a fact that 95% of all balding or bald men suffer from male pattern baldness. Male pattern baldness usually starts with a receding hairline at the front and is frequently accompanied with thinning at the top.

Over time, this thinning turns into a full-fledged bald spot, and the bald spot grows to cover the head, apart from the sides and around the back.

Regardless of this, as long as there is a single hair left on my head I'll still demand a stylish coiffure. So, what balding hairstyle options are available?

1. The worst balding men's hairstyle is the **comb over**. This is the classic look belonging to men of a certain age whereby the hair is grown longer on one side of the head and 'combed over' the bald area to the other side.

This strategy simply spells disaster even in the slightest of breezes and is to be avoided at all costs.

Don'ts

But assuming you already know this, what are the other dos and don'ts to balding men's hairstyles?

- The first common mistake is combing the hair straight back. This may cover bald spots, but it only exposes the forehead and draws attention to the receding hairline.

- The second is growing your hair longer at the back to make up for what's lacking on top. This unbalances the head and draws even more attention to the scalp and the baldness.
- Younger men with thinning hair might be tempted to use gel… but this isn't recommended. Gel clumps your hair together and reveals the scalp.
- Likewise, growing your hair long in an attempt to cover up actually causes hair to separate and show more scalp.

So, what are the dos?

- Get more natural looking fluff to your hair by using mousses and conditioners.
- Grow your remaining hair by a few inches, get it layered and brush it forward to break up the receding hairline.
- If your hairline isn't receding too badly, but the top of your head is thinning, you can get away with keeping the front long and combing your hair straight back to cover the bald spot. Eventually however, your bald spot will expand.

2. The ultimate balding men's hairstyle when faced with a shiny bald dome, is to go the whole hog and shave it off or at least a very close trim. You'll probably be amazed at people's reactions and the compliments you'll get – the shaved look is a totally acceptable balding hairstyle these days.

Steps to follow

- Start with electric clippers like you'll find in the barbers. After you've clipped the heavy stuff, lather up with shaving gel. This gives you a closer, smoother shave than shaving cream.
- Then using a razor, start at the top and shave down with the grain taking care at the back. It's recommended to watch what you're doing with a small mirror.

Care for a Shaved Head

Shaving your head only takes a few minutes and you don't need to do it every day (two to three times a week is fine). Taking care of your new shaved head is much like taking care of your face. Wash regularly with moisturizing soap, rather than a harsh deodorant soap that can dry out the skin on your head. Also use a good quality moisturizer after every wash – cheaper moisturizers will just clog up your pores.

For the summer, find a moisturizer with a sun protection factor of at least 15 to avoid sunburn on your head. And you'll need a warm hat in winter to maintain your body heat.

If shaving doesn't tickle your fancy then you can always opt for a hairpiece as a last resort - though I wouldn't recommend it :-)

Chapter Six

HAIR DISORDERS

Trichotillomania

Keywords: *causes of trichotillomania, Telogen effluvium, Tinea capitis*

Abstract: *It looks strange to find someone pulling out his/her hair under the influence of an uncontrollable urge. Some may call it madness, or witchcraft, but it's a hair disorder.*

What is Trichotillomania?

The term "trichotillomania" comes from the Greek words "thrix," meaning "hair" and "tillein" meaning "to pull" and "mania," the Greek word for "madness" or "frenzy". As the name suggests trichotillomania is a psychiatric condition in which an individual has an uncontrollable urge to pull out his or her own body hair. For people suffering from trichotillomania, hair pulling is more than a habit. It is rather a compulsive behavior, which the person finds very hard to stop. The cause of trichotillomania is supposed to be the imbalance of chemicals in the human brain.

People with trichotillomania pull their hair out of the root from places like the scalp, eyebrows, eyelashes, or even the pubic area (ouch!). Some people even pull handfuls of hair, which can leave bald patches on the scalp or eyebrows. Other people pull out their hair one strand at a time. Some inspect the strands after pulling them out or play with the hair after it's been pulled. About half of the people with this condition also have the habit of putting the plucked hair in their mouth.

Trichotillomania has been mentioned as a disorder in very early historical records. But clinically the condition trichotillomania was first described in 1889 by the French physician Francois

Hallopeau. The condition is rare - statistics show it affects only 1% to 3% of the population, although new research suggests that the rate of hair pulling may be around 10% or higher.

Who is More Affected, Male or Female?

Trichotillomania affects about twice as many girls as boys. Most people who have trichotillomania develop the condition during adolescence. However, it can start when a person is as young as 1 year old.

Effects of Trichotillomania

Trichotillomania is often the cause of embarrassment, frustration, shame, or depression for those people affected with the disorder. Those people also suffer from low self-esteem. They usually try to hide their behavior from others. Because of this fact, social alienation is common in trichotillomania patients. Moreover, the patients also try to cover patches of balding scalp by wearing wigs, hats, scarves or hair clips, or by applying make-up or even by tattooing.

Causes of Trichotillomania

Doctors don't know much about the cause of trichotillomania. It is believed that genetics plays a major role. The compulsive behavior like trichotillomania can sometimes run in families. Some psychiatrists think it might be related to OCD since OCD and trichotillomania are both anxiety disorders. This is one reason why the impulses that lead to hair pulling can be stronger when a person is stressed out or worried.

Experts think that the actual cause of trichotillomania is the imbalance of chemicals in the brain. These chemicals, called **neurotransmitters** are part of the brain's communication center. When something interferes with how neurotransmitters work it can cause problems like compulsive behaviors.

Since trichotillomania is a medical condition, it's not something most people can just stop doing when they feel like it. People with trichotillomania usually need help from medical experts before they can stop. With the right help, though, most people overcome their hair-pulling urges. This help may involve

- Therapy
- Medication, or a combination of both.

There are therapies in which special behavior techniques are used to help people recognize the urge to pull hair before the urge becomes too strong to resist. The patient learns ways to resist the urge so that the urge becomes weaker and then goes away.

Many people find it helpful to keep their hands busy with a different activity (like squeezing a stress ball or drawing) during times when the urge of pulling hair is strong. Even activities like knitting while watching TV seems to help.

CHAPTER SEVEN

HAIR LOSS TREATMENTS

Are Hair Loss Treatments Just One Big Scam?

The hair loss industry has attracted a lot of criticism over the years. But is this fully justified or are there some genuine ways to deal with premature baldness?

The hair loss treatments industry is not one that inspires great confidence in most people. I have to admit this is perfectly understandable given the damage caused by the many rogues and charlatans who have abused the trust of far too many vulnerable people - people who have received worthless and even dangerous products or advice in exchange for their hard earned cash. The end result is the prevalence of a stigma that the industry is hard pressed to shake off.

But is this perception really justified nowadays? Are there no genuine treatments that sufferers can turn to in a bid to treat the ravages of premature hair loss? The simple answer is YES, there are several safe, affordable, accessible and effective hair loss treatments currently available. Some have even been approved by FDA for the treatment of hair loss conditions while others draw on natural remedies as the basis for commercially available products. Whether or not any of them are suitable for a given individual depends on a number of important factors.

First and foremost, every individual must determine the exact cause or causes of his or her hair loss. This may appear to be an over-simplistic statement but the truth is, most people undergoing a course of treatment for hair loss have proceeded on the basis of self-diagnosis. Given the fact that premature or excessive hair loss is often associated with underlying medical conditions, this is perhaps not the most sensible course of action.

My advice in all cases is to seek the guidance of a qualified medical practitioner because the consequences of not doing so may be serious in a small number of cases. Even where all the evidence points to the onset of hereditary male pattern baldness it would probably be best to seek advice, if only to rule out other factors.

Once the cause of hair loss has been properly diagnosed you will be in a position to choose a suitable form of treatment. This may range from the prescription of drugs aimed at balancing disrupted hormone levels to the topical application of *minoxidil* to reduce the symptoms of male pattern baldness.

Hair loss may be caused by many factors including

- Changing hormone levels
- Stress
- Overuse of strong chemicals
- Excessive traction
- Poor grooming practices
- Side effects of medical treatment
- Weak immune system and
- Aging
- Autoimmune disorders
- Diseases
- Nutritional deficiencies
- Poisons
- Prescription drugs
- Chemotherapy drugs
- Radiation exposure
- Physical trauma to the scalp
- Hair loss following childbirth
- Psychological
- Hair styling techniques
- Hair styling products

The good news is, all of these can be tackled with reasonable hope of success but only if you choose the right treatment.

The next e-book in this series will look closely at the various causes of excessive hair loss and outline suggested treatments that are both affordable and accessible. If you will take only two things from this section, please take these suggestions on board:

1. Always seek the advice of your physician before undergoing a hair loss treatment regime.

2. Don't despair, there's often a simple explanation for excessive hair loss and even hereditary loss or male pattern-type baldness can be treated successfully for most people nowadays.

Topical Hair Loss Treatments

If you are a man, it is quite common that you may experience some hair loss in your lifetime. Many men lose hair when they are in their twenties; some are a little luckier and lose their hair in their late forties. If you have noticed that you have lost your hair, there are a couple of treatments available. Here are some tips.

Hair loss is very common, however it is very difficult for many men to deal with. Hair loss can affect a person's looks and self-esteem. If you are losing your hair there are two main treatments that have been proven effective. They are topical treatments and a drug that works via pill form.

Topical treatments include *Rogaine*, which has the effective ingredient *Minoxodil*. *Minoxodil* has been proven effective, but does not grow your entire hair back. Depending on where the loss of hair is located, you can see some moderate regrowth from *Minoxodil*. *Minoxodil* is a solution that is topical; you apply it to your scalp twice a day. It is usually inexpensive, costing about $20 per month.

Propecia is a pill that can be taken by men experiencing hair loss; it is proven effective and usually works better than *Minoxodil*. You take the pill once a day and can significantly regrow your hair or slow down how much hair you lose. However it is not a miracle drug and won't regrow all your hair back. So if you are losing your hair, look into these two possible treatments.

More information can be found at http://www.health-00.info/hair-loss/

The Search for the Best Hair Loss Treatment Product

Keywords: Best hair loss treatment product,

Abstract: Here we give you a tour of the many hair loss treatment products available to you, giving enough information on each to enable you to decide which ones you will try in order to cure your hair loss problem.

Googling the Best Hair Loss Treatment Product

You have probably asked yourself time and time again, what is the best hair loss treatment product available? That question was asked on a Google answers site, and the experts answer? They stated that there is no answer to that question.

They are correct in that there is no general answer to that question, but there is an answer to the alternative question, "What is the best hair loss treatment product for me?" It's still not an easy question to answer though, and you'll probably need to find the answer via good old-fashioned trial and error methods.

Is Home Remedies The Best Hair Treatment Product?

There are many kinds of home remedies for hair loss. I'm pretty sure some of them can be disregarded — like rubbing cow manure on your head — but some of them probably do help some people. Here are a few of the more promising home remedies for hair loss:

- Rinse your hair with *apple cider vinegar* and *sage tea*.
- A variety of oils have been used—*almond oil, castor oil, olive oil*, and *amla oil*. Usually the oil is warmed, which will at least feel good and make your hair shiny.
- Applying coconut milk or *Aloe vera* gel to your scalp.

- Applying a masque of honey and egg yolk to your hair and scalp.

All of these concoctions should be washed out (except the apple cider and sage tea rinse) after use.

Is It Hair Care Products?

The best hair loss treatment product for you could be as simple as a good shampoo or conditioner. Some people swear by *Nizoral* shampoo, and say it puts an end to hair loss. Some people love *Mane and Tail* shampoo and conditioner, because it makes their hair look and feel fuller and thicker. Your hairdresser may have some suggestions about hair care products that help you with your hair loss

Or Herbal Remedies?

Some people believe that the best hair loss treatment product is an herbal remedy. There are a number of herbal lotions and potions as well as nutritional supplements specially formulated to treat hair loss. An herbalist may be able to recommend the best products for your particular type of hair loss. Here are a few herbal remedies that seem to help:

- Ginko biloba
- Green tea
- Chinese herb called "He Shou Wu"
- Pygeum
- Aloe vera
- Saw palmetto
- Stinging nettle

Some of these are taken in pill form and some are made into preparations that you rub onto your scalp. Some (like, for instance, stinging nettles) can cause a reaction, so use all herbal preparations with care.

What about Minoxidil (Rogain®)?

A lot of people consider that this is the best hair loss treatment product. It's available without a prescription at any pharmacy, and it works for a lot of people. Minoxidil helps both men and women to grow more hair. Remember, though, that as soon as you quit taking minoxidil, your hair will start to fall out again.

Prescription Medications?

A prescription medication, such as *Propecia*, could be the ideal hair loss treatment product for you. You need to see the doctor to get it, but that's a good thing, because she will conduct a check-up to see if there is some underlying cause to your hair loss that can be taken care of permanently.

Wigs, Rugs or Weaves?

It could turn to be that the best hair loss treatment product for you is a cover up of some kind. This is especially true when the hair loss is temporary, such as when your hair falls out while undergoing chemotherapy.

There are a lot of options available to you to treat hair loss, but only you can decide which one is the best hair loss treatment product for you. Test a few things, and when you find something that works for you, stick with it. It may not work for everybody, but the important thing here is that you will have found the best hair loss treatment product for you.

How to Identify the Best Hair Loss Treatment Products

Keywords: *Best Hair loss treatment products, Hair loss help, Hair loss prevention, hair loss cure, hair loss, hair care, hair loss solution.*

Abstract: *This chapter 'How to Identify the Best Hair loss treatment product' is helpful to those men / women who are going bald. After reading this chapter you will be able to identify your hair problems and this will help you as well as others to prevent hair loss. This will help in developing a healthy society.*

Is there a 100% Hair Loss Treatment Product?

Our society is becoming bald; you can find a bald person in every nook and corner of your locality. You don't need to search, if you are the one. Hair loss is a deficiency that can make any person bald. Earlier, it was the men, now it is affecting the women also in equal proportion. Sometime children also suffer from hair loss. In fact, hair loss is a natural phenomenon and also happens as biological clock ticks but if this clock ticks frequently, then it is called a deficiency, the baldness. This might happen because of improper nutrition, low hygiene, various environmental circumstances etc.

"One's loss is others gain;" the saying goes well in case of baldness too.

A number of products are available in the market to prevent hair loss and they are labelled "100% guarantee" But if this has been the case, then today it would be difficult to find any man / women with hair loss problems in the area you live, because these hair loss treatment products have been existing in the market for decades and the public is buying and trying the different products to stay hairy. The person who has hair on their head and shaves it is another side of the story. The hair loss treatment products claim them to be medically proven and people are trying these products with no success at all. I'm sure if you are one of them you definitely have tried some of these products. Since you have tried the product, do you have any idea about hair loss treatment products? You will definitely say NO. This is because one product, which may be good for one person, may be a dump for another and vice-versa.

In most of the hair loss cases it has been found that the hair loss treatment products recommended by a physician gave better results. That's why, hair loss today is not merely the baldness but a type of sickness which need to be checked, diagnosed and treated by an expert physician rather than going for trial and error treatments, using one hair loss treatment product today, another tomorrow, and so on, which may be of no result. So, if you are suffering hair loss problems, you need to identify the source of your hair loss problems and see your physician, and get the problem solved.

Clinical diagnosis of hair loss patients suggests that in most of the cases, the reason for hair loss was improper diet, a deficiency of different vitamins and minerals in the body, stress, side effects of medications for any particular sickness, irregular sleep, etc. So, it is obvious that if you are suffering from hair loss or someone around you is and you want to help the person, then try to identify the origin of the problem of hair loss and take the good medical help of experts rather than trying products available in the store shelves.

Sometime a person suffering hair loss may opt for herbal hair loss treatment products, because it is believed that herbal remedies causes no or minimal side effects. If you are affected, and thinking to buy some herbal hair loss treatment product then make sure that the product you are going to try will restore dead hair follicles and support hair growth. But at the same time remember that these herbal remedies may have side effects, so it is best and most favorable to go for your doctors' advice before trying any herbal hair loss treatment product as well.

NOTE: Women be cautious if you are suffering hair loss. Never use any hair loss treatment product without getting an expert advice. Some of the hair loss treatment products may cause growth of hair all over the body and definitely you don't want hair on your upper lips (that will be awful)

Therefore, it is best for both sexes to take precaution, and try only products recommended by a qualified doctor. You also need to understand the causes of hair loss, so that you can help yourself and others to minimize the chances of hair loss / baldness or prevent it.

The following things are what you need to understand to prevent your hair problems:

- The ways to either prevent or stop hair loss and the knowledge of promoting hair growth.

- The ways to increase the lifespan of hair cells and promote follicles growth.

- The several internal and external factors that also affect your hair health and promote hair problems like thinning hairs etc. Knowing these factors and having the knowledge of hair and scalp rejuvenation.

- Some cosmetic products also may harm your hair, so if you have opted for some new product and you are experiencing some problems, switch it over, immediately. Go for your old brand. After all *'old is gold'*.

- Know the diet and lifestyle that will suit your hair too.

- Know the methods of improving hair longevity.

- Hair loss in some cases is genetic. Knowing the facts and how to minimize it will help a lot.

- Hair loss is equally common amongst women, so women should also know the causes and cure of it.

- Stress, high blood pressure and heart disease also leads to hair loss. Knowing these facts and trying to get more knowledge about it will be of great help.

Herbs for Hair Loss Treatment

Every human being experiences hair loss at some time in their lives. It is very rare that any one does not suffer it. If you are one of those who are losing hair, please read the complete e-book. In this chapter, you are advised the best hair loss treatment.

Scientifically Proven Herbs for Hair Loss Treatment:

The following herbs have been scientifically proven and testified to have remarkable efficacy as hair loss treatments:

   *Carya alba*

   *Astragalus glycyphyllos*

   *Angelica arhangelica* Root

   Peach Kernel Oil

   Alvia *officinalis*

   *Capsicum*

   Cortex D*ictamni radicis*

   Flos *chrysanthemum*

   *Heshouwu*

   Iron-Fist *Ginseng*

   *Miltiorrhizae*

   *Notoginseng*

   *Paorulca glandulosa*

   *Rhizome of Szechuan Lovage*

   *Radix astragali*

   *Radix GinsengRadix Polygoni Multiflori*

   *Corthamis tinctorius*

   *Red-rooted Salvia*

   *Aralia quinquetolia*

   *Rhizhoma gastroidia ginseng*

   *Seu radix notopterygii*

   *Sophera flavescens*

The Best Hair Loss Treatment Products are:

- 101D Hair Loss Treatment
- 101F Hair Loss Treatment

- 101G Hair Loss Treatment and
- 101 Hair Loss Treatment Shampoo

The above are the names of hair loss treatment products which are regarded as the best hair loss treatment products by world renowned hair experts. These products not only include the aforementioned important herbs for hair loss treatment, but also include them in the molecular structure that is vital for highly effective hair loss recovery.

Use of these products according to the given directions will help you achieve:

- Thickness and beauty in existing hair
- Scalp and follicle conditions that is improved
- Noticeable hair re-growth
- Low rate of hair loss

Best Hair Loss Treatment - A Lot of Options

Keywords: Hair Loss treatments, hair loss, hair loss remedy, hair care, hair fall, baldness

Abstract: Hair loss creates baldness. A bald person looks older than his real age. This abnormal hair loss is technically called alopecia. It does not affect your health directly but indirectly it creates problems, such as low self-esteem. When alopecia occurs at a young age, it creates an inferiority complex that leads to other health problems. Hence, we should attend to this problem and go for a hair loss treatment. There are many treatments; some are medications and some are surgeries.

Hair loss creates baldness.

A bald person looks older than his real age. This abnormal hair loss is technically called alopecia. It does not affect your health directly but indirectly it creates problems, such as low self-esteem. When alopecia occurs at a young age, it creates an inferiority complex that leads to other health problems. Hence, we should attend to this problem and go for a hair loss treatment. There are many treatments; some are medications and some are surgeries. You need to find the best hair loss treatment by consulting a specialist. If the condition is not severe, then, you can stop the hair loss with **Propecia**.

Propecia is a well-known medicine and very popular. A regular use of Propecia can stop hair loss and even re-grow hair. Not just Propecia, there are other options too that could be better for your hair. In the past people did not have many options to fight baldness. The most common way was to buy a wig and cover the head. But now with the advancement of science we have many more ways for treating hair loss. Some of the better hair loss treatments are:

- **Bio matrix treatment**: This is widely known as hair weaving. Hair is woven to cover the bald patch. Today hair weaving has emerged as one of the best and popular treatments for hair loss.
- **Surgical hair transplant**: The hair follicles in the bald patches are transplanted with hair. In each follicle up to four hairs can be transplanted. Hair is picked from other areas of your scalp where hair is still thick. To be successful this treatment needs a healthy growth.

These are some of the well-known hair loss treatments that are famous and widely used. A lot of people have been benefited by these treatments.

Paul has been providing answers to lots of queries through his website on a wide variety of subjects ranging from satellite phones to acne.

Best Male Hair Loss Treatment Products

Keywords: *Hair loss treatment product, Stop hair loss, Rogaine, Order Rogaine, Propecia, Hair loss treatment, Hair loss*

Abstract: *The worse part of getting older is joint aches and loss of hair. Chances of getting bald are more if you are a male and your age is more than 45. Alopecia or male pattern baldness is genetic in character. Medical hair transplants are used by many people every year with surprising results to overcome this problem. But hair transplant is the last solution of hair loss problem. Some hair loss remedies are available in the market for hair loss prevention. Moreover, you can stop.*

Maleness and Hair Loss

The worse part of getting older is joint aches and loss of hair. Chances of getting bald are more if you are a male and your age is more than 45. Alopecia or male pattern baldness is genetic in character. Medical hair transplants are used by many people every year with surprising results to overcome this problem. But hair transplant is the last solution of hair loss problem. Some hair loss remedies are available in the market for hair loss prevention. Moreover, you can stop hair loss with the use of best hair loss treatment products (allopathic). With the use of hair loss treatment products, you can simply stop hair loss, no new hair loss will occur.

Alopecia or male pattern baldness is not a scalp related problem. Alopecia occurs as a result of chemical reaction between oil glands found in the hair follicle and testosterone. When testosterone (male hormone) transforms into DHT, reaction causes follicle to shrink. But there are hair loss treatment products available on the market, which works against the production of DHT. You must buy a hair loss treatment product, which contains ingredients like ***Pro-vitamin B5***, ***Saw*** and ***Palmetto Zinc***. These kinds of hair loss treatment product are designed to keep your hair on your head.

If you want to stop hair loss, you are recommended to use hair loss treatment products like ***Propecia*** and ***Rogaine***. These hair loss treatment products are available at drug stores and you can even order Rogaine online. If it is already late and you are bald or have significant thinning, then you must think of a hair loss treatment. Medical hair restoration will be the best option for your problem. Results will be full head of natural hair. This process is not painful, but you will feel some swelling and discomfort. Your dermatologist will help you select a hair loss treatment product or hair transplant process, which will meet your expectations.

CHAPTER EIGHT

UNDERSTANDING DHT

DHT BLOCKER

Keywords: *Natural DHT Blocker, Best DHT Blocker, DHT Blocker, Procerin, Male Hair Loss.*

Abstract: *DHT Blocker supplements have to be taken on a regular basis twice a day as a preventive measure, though the kind of DHT blocker supplement depends on the cause of the high level of DHT in the body.*

Natural DHT Blocker

DHT is now widely believed to be the devil behind the problem of hair loss. Over ninety five percent of hair loss cases are the cause of DHT and so the main course of action in treating DHT is to stop it by using a (http://www.dhtblocker.net/dht-blocker-natural.html) natural DHT blocker.

There are many ways to accomplish blocking of DHT and these include keeping DHT from attaching to the receptors of the hair follicles, reducing the production of DHT in the first place, inhibiting the production of the enzyme 5 alpha reductase, the main cause for the existence of DHT or reduce the substance that produces the enzyme 5 alpha reductase - cholesterol. A (http://www.dhtblocker.net/) DHT blocker is any substance that can produce any of the conditions mentioned here. Once DHT is effectively blocked the remaining hair follicles will be able to convalesce and begin to grow healthy hair once again.

Nature: The best Physician

Zinc: The best natural DHT blocker is **Zinc**. Zinc is freely available in nature and natural foods rich in zinc will help in blocking DHT naturally.

Saw palmetto. In-depth research of this natural DHT blocker reveal that *Saw palmetto* is a very effective natural DHT blocker and acts very similarly to **Propecia** by firstly lowering the DHT in the body by effectively blocking the 5 *alpha-reductase* and then by blocking the receptor sites on cell membranes that absorb DHT. This is by far the most convenient way to block DHT naturally.

DHT also contributes to other diseases of the body such as prostate cancer. So, (http://www.Procerin.com/) hair loss is not the only problem brought on by DHT in the body. All of the studies that have been performed to date show that Saw palmetto is an effective anti-androgen and has shown conclusively to be effective in the treatment of benign prostratic disease as well as killing off of the hair follicles in the body. *Saw palmetto* is a very potent natural DHT blocker.

Pygeum extract is another natural DHT blocker that inhibit the production of DHT in the body. *Pygeum* has been proven to have ingredients that effectively reduce prolacting levels and block the accumulation of cholesterol in the prostate glands. Prolactin is also believed to increase the uptake of testosterone by the prostate, and cholesterol increases binding sites for DHT. *Pygeum* basically reduces the levels of DHT in the blood and reduces the number of sites where DHT can attach thus is also a very effective way to naturally reduce DHT levels. Pay a visit to www.Procerin.com and get firsthand information on all the ways to reduce DHT levels naturally. You will emerge all the wiser and ready to face the problem better when next you confer with your doctor.

DHT Blocker Supplement

Keywords: *DHT Blocker Supplements, Herbal Supplements, Best DHT Blocker, DHT Blocker, Procerin.*

Abstract: *DHT Blocker supplements have to be taken on a regular basis twice a day as a preventive measure, though the kind of DHT blocker supplement depends on the cause of the high level of DHT in the body.*

Do Hair Supplements Really Work?

People read e-books and ads of hair loss supplements in almost every publication everyday. These are herbal supplements and steroid based hair loss supplement but do these Hair Loss supplements really work? Most of the hair loss is caused by DHT or Dihydrotestosterone. This is a naturally occurring enzyme, and one of the most potent ones in the human body, and is produced by the reaction of an enzyme called 5 alpha-reductase with the hormone testosterone; this DHT is the main cause of thinning of hair which finally leads to hair loss in men and women.

When DHT formed by the 5 alpha-reductase enzyme reacts with testosterone in the fair follicles, the DHT thus formed attaches itself to the receptor cells of the air follicle thus stifling the growth of the hair. This finally leads to loss of hair because the DHT finally kills the hair follicle. Luckily for many, this condition can be reversed or rather prevented by taking DHT Blocker Supplements that stop or block DHT formation in the body. These can be herbal supplements or laboratory prepared steroids with the ability to stop the effects of DHT and finally assist the re growth of hair in men between the ages of eighteen and forty. However, whatever the DHT blocker supplements one is advised to take them only in consultancy with a qualified medical practitioner as some of the DHT blocker supplements have serious side effects.

How long does one wait to see results?

DHT Blocker supplements have to be taken on a regular basis twice a day as a preventive measure, though the kind of DHT blocker supplement depends on the cause of the high level of DHT in the body. The results of DHT blocker supplements can be seen in the first week of taking the DHT blocker supplements. The improvements continue over the next six or eight weeks. One pack of DHT Blocker supplements lasts for a month though you will find some good advice and offers on Procerin.

Some of the better known DHT blocker supplements are *Saw Palmetto* or *Serenoa repens*. The berries of these naturally available DHT blocker supplements contain certain fatty acids and sterols that effectively block 5-Alpha-Reductase and reduce DHT uptake by hair follicles thus preventing hair loss very effectively. The other DHT blocker supplements are *Boarage oil*, *Stinging nettle* or *Urtica diocia* and *Green tea* as well as *grape seed extract*. For a greater description of how these DHT blocker supplements can help you click here http://www.dhtblocker.net/dht-blocker-supplement.html

CHAPTER NINE

HAIR CARE AND OTHER THINGS

Chemicals in Shampoo May Pose Health Risks

Keywords: *Chemicals in Shampoo May Pose Health Risks*

Abstract: *Have you ever read the label on your shampoo bottle? You'll be shocked to learn that the ingredients found in many shampoos may pose a threat to your health.*

Compositions of a Shampoo

Have you ever read the label on your shampoo bottle? You'll be shocked to learn that the ingredients found in many shampoos may pose a threat to your health. Research has shown that various chemicals lurking inside shampoo may induce serious health risks, like memory loss, eye and skin irritation, hair follicle damage that can lead to hair loss, and even cancer.

While the U.S. Food and Drug Administration classifies personal care products, it does not regulate them. Therefore, there are no legal guidelines or boundaries for shampoo manufacturers to follow.

The descriptive "all-natural" has become a buzzword in the beauty world for environmental friendliness. What some shampoo makers leave out, however, is they still use the lathering agents, emulsifiers and synthetic fragrances that contain hundreds of harmful chemicals.

According to a company called Blinc Inc., it is very likely that the list of ingredients in a bottle of shampoo will contain some of the following additives:

- **Propylene glycol** known as the main ingredient in antifreeze, is also found in makeup, toothpaste and in your shampoo. It can cause allergic reactions.

- **Sodium lauryl sulfate** and ammonium lauryl sulfate are common causes of eye irritation. They can also damage hair follicles. When absorbed into the body from continuous contact, they can bring on asthma attacks.

- **Synthetic fragrances** contain hundreds of chemicals, some of which have been known to cause headaches, dizziness, rash, hyperpigmentation, coughing and vomiting.

- **Diethanolamine**: The National Toxicology Program found that applying diethanolamine (DEA) to a mouse's skin induced liver and kidney cancer. DEA is readily absorbed through the skin and can also be toxic to the brain.

But before you decide to never wash your hair again, Blinc Inc. is simplifying consumer education by consolidating official government research on questionable ingredients found in many shampoos, conditioners and body washes.

The company's philosophy of "Why take a chance?" means there are no controversial ingredients in its haircare products. They are 99.8 percent vegetable derived and as close to natural as possible while effectively cleansing without causing irritation to eyes or skin or damaging hair.

Dandruff - Are You Sure It's Dandruff?

Keywords: Dandruff, hair, skin, eczema, psoriasis

Abstract: Everybody hates dandruff. Nobody likes the falling white flakes and the itching scalp. We all try many shampoos and treatments, both natural and chemical to get rid of dandruff. I want to ask many of you who suffer dandruff- how are you sure that you are having dandruff? Unless a doctor diagnosed it as dandruff, how can anyone be sure that he/she is suffering

dandruff if it is not clearing after many washes? May be you are suffering from something else?
Let us look at the other problems that may confuse you.

Identifying Dandruff

Everybody hates dandruff. Nobody likes the falling white flakes and the itching scalp. We all try many shampoos and treatments, both natural and chemical to get rid of dandruff. I want to ask many of you who suffer dandruff- how are you sure that you are having dandruff? Unless a doctor diagnosed it as dandruff, how can anyone be sure that he/she is suffering dandruff if it is not clearing after many washes? May be you are suffering from something else? Let us look at the other problems that may confuse you.

Dandruff and other scalp problems

There are many scalp problems that itch and produce scales and white flakes. ***Psoriasis*** is one of the tough ones. Unless you get it diagnosed and get treated it will not go away. Many cosmetic applications may cause allergic dermatitis or irritant contact dermatitis. Atopic dermatitis or commonly called ***eczema*** can also appear on the scalp. Seborrheic dermatitis is one of the common scalp problems that mimic dandruff.

What is dandruff?

In dandruff, what we see as white flakes are skin cells. Our skin regenerates itself every month. The new cells travel from the bottom of the skin layer to the top in a month and the dead cells are shed. These are so microscopic and small in quantity that we don't notice this shedding of cells. In dandruff this shedding increases. That is how these dead cells with skin oils form white flakes and we can see them.

Dandruff and diagnosis

If you are not able to get rid of dandruff after trying many formulas, it is time that you visit a doctor and get the proper diagnosis done. Once you are sure that it is dandruff, you can take proper measures and get a shiny scalp.

This e-book is only for informative purposes. This e-book is not intended to be a medical advice and it is not a substitute for professional medical advice. Please consult your doctor for your medical concerns. Please follow any tip given in this e-book only after consulting your doctor. The author is not liable for any outcome or damage resulting from information obtained from this e-book.

Dandruff - What Causes Dandruff?

Dandruff is one of the most common scalp problems. But it is surprising that no precise cause off dandruff is known. There is therefore no cure for dandruff, but you can treat it whenever it shows. There are many factors that trigger dandruff and some speculation about the possible causes. Let us talk about them so that we can keep our scalp squeaky clean from dandruff.

Dandruff and fungus

Dandruff is a kind of Seborrheic dermatitis and it is believed that dandruff is caused by a fungus that normally lives on the human skin and feeds on skin oils. During dandruff, this fungus known as malassezia multiplies manifold and creates problems in the scalp. Why a fungus, which otherwise lies dormant, suddenly flares up and multiplies is not precisely known.

Dandruff and other causes

Other causes that are held responsible for dandruff are:

- Stress
- Poor hygiene of scalp
- Over use of shampoos

- Under use of shampoo

- Chemical treatments that harm the hair and scalp etc.

The incidence of dandruff is less in summer than in winter. We can deduce that less sun may be causing dandruff, but exposing ourselves more to the sun may cause serious skin problems.